Abortion in Asia

ABORTION IN ASIA
Local Dilemmas, Global Politics

Edited by
Andrea Whittaker

Berghahn Books
New York • Oxford

FOUNDATION®
BOOKS

Delhi • Bengaluru • Mumbai • Kolkata • Chennai • Hyderabad
Pune • Thiruvananthapuram

Published by
Cambridge University Press India Pvt. Ltd.
under the imprint of Foundation Books
Cambridge House, 4381/4 Ansari Road, Daryaganj, **New Delhi** 110 002

Cambridge University Press India Pvt. Ltd.
C-22, C-Block, Brigade M.M., K.R. Road, Jayanagar, **Bengaluru** 560 070
Plot No. 80, Service Industries, Shirvane, Sector-1, Nerul, **Navi Mumbai** 400 706
10 Raja Subodh Mullick Square, 2nd Floor, **Kolkata** 700 013
21/1 (New No. 49), 1st Floor, Model School Road, Thousand Lights, **Chennai** 600 006
House No. 3-5-874/6/4, (Near Apollo Hospital), Hyderguda, **Hyderabad** 500 029
Agarwal Pride, 'A' Wing, 1308 Kasba Peth, Near Surya Hospital, **Pune** 411 011
T.C. 25/ 2731 Lukes Lane, Ambujavilasam Road, **Thiruvananthapuram** 695 001

This edition is published by Cambridge University Press India Pvt. Ltd. by arrangement with Berghahn Books Ltd.

First South Asia Edition 2014

ISBN 978-93-82993-15-5

Published by Manas Saikia for Cambridge University Press India Pvt. Ltd. and printed at Bhavish Graphics, Chennai

Contents

Figures

Illustrations

Tables

Documents

Acknowledgements

This book could not have been written without the participation of the many women and men who volunteered their stories to the authors. For many it would have been the first time they gave accounts of their abortions. Our sincere thanks for their time and trust.

This work was inspired by my initial research on abortion in Thailand which was supported by a Discovery Project grant of the Australian Research Council. I am grateful to all the authors in this volume who patiently suffered initial delays to this project and responded to my endless requests with good humour, and thanks also to the various organisations that support them. I also wish to thank Katerina Aleksoska and Aren Aizura who assisted with the editing and formatting of the manuscript. I greatly appreciated their advice and dedication to the task.

I am indebted to my husband Bruce Missingham for his ceaseless encouragement, critical reviews and thoughtful advice, and to my two daughters, Claire and Rachel, for delaying the manuscript in the most delightful ways. This book is dedicated to advocates striving for reproductive rights across Asia.

CONTRIBUTORS

Rashidah Abdullah is a researcher and activist and core founder of a number of women's NGOs including Sisters in Islam (1989), The Asian-Pacific Resource and Research Centre for Women (ARROW) in 1993, The Global Forum for Health Research (Geneva) in 1997 and the Reproductive Rights Advocacy Alliance Malaysia (RRAAM) in 2006 of which she is Co-Chair.

Dr Suzanne Belton is a Senior Lecturer at the Menzies School of Health Research, Darwin. Her current research interests include Australian Indigenous women's experiences of the maternity system in the Northern Territory, maternal mortality in Timor-Leste and post-abortion care.

Nongluk Boonthai formerly worked at the Reproductive Health Division, Department of Health, Ministry of Public Health, Thailand. She now works at the Women's Health and Reproductive Rights Foundation of Thailand (WHRRF).

Professor Kamheang Chaturachinda is a founder of the Women's Health and Reproductive Rights Foundation of Thailand (WHRRF). He was former President of the Royal Thai College of Obstetricians and Gynecologists (RTCOG).

Dr Tine Gammeltoft is an Associate Professor, Department of Anthropology, University of Copenhagen, Denmark.

Dr Elizabeth Hoban is a Senior Lecturer, School of Health and Social Development, Deakin University, Melbourne.

Amanda Huber is former Asia Programs Associate at Ipas, Chapel Hill, North Carolina, and is currently consulting in health economics and policy.

Terence Hull is Adjunct Professor of Demography in the Australian Demographic and Social Research Institute, The Australian National University, Canberra, Australia.

Alyson Hyman is Senior Advisor in the Training and Service Delivery Improvement Unit at Ipas, Chapel Hill, North Carolina.

Professor Pertti J. Pelto is retired Professor Emeritus at the University of Connecticut.

Dr Lam Phirun is Senior Programme Coordinator for the National Reproductive Health Programme, Ministry of Health, Cambodia.

Dr Lakshmi Ramachandar is an independent researcher in India, who has carried out extensive research concerning abortion in Tamil Nadu, Karnataka, and Jharkhand states.

Dr Sabina Faiz Rashid is Co-ordinator at the Centre for Gender, Sexuality and HIV/AIDS at the James P. Grant School of Public Health, BRAC University, Dhaka, Bangladesh.

Dr Tung Rathavy is the Programme Manager for the National Reproductive Health Programme, Ministry of Health, Cambodia.

Dr. Viroj Tangcharoensathien is Director of International Health Policy Program in the Ministry of Public Health, Thailand. His recent work includes the design of the Social Health Insurance and Universal Coverage Scheme in Thailand.

Dr Sripen Tantivess specializes in health policy analysis and works in the Health Intervention and Technology Assessment Program and the International Health Policy Program, Ministry of Public Health, Thailand.

Dr Phan Bich Thuy is former Senior Training & Services Advisor for Ipas, located in Hanoi, Vietnam, and currently an international reproductive health consultant.

Dr Andrea Whittaker is Associate Professor and ARC Future Fellow, Social Sciences and Health Unit, School of Psychology and Psychiatry, Monash University, Melbourne, Australia. Her previous work included an ethnography on abortion in rural Thailand (2004). Her current research interests include work on infertility and reproductive tourism in Thailand and the region.

Ninuk Widyantoro is the Founder of *Yayasan Kesehatan Perempuan* (Women's Health Foundation) Jakarta, Indonesia.

Merrill Wolf is Senior Advisor for Strategic Partnerships at Ipas, Chapel Hill, North Carolina.

Dr Yut-Lin Wong, an Associate Professor at the Department of Social and Preventive Medicine, Faculty of Medicine, University of Malaya, is an activist researcher in sexual reproductive health and rights, and gender-based violence. As advocate for women's rights, she is involved in several women's NGOs engaged in the national campaign against violence against women.

Chapter One

Abortion in Asia

An overview

Andrea Whittaker

Aunty Phim

At my age [forty-five years old] it's not normal [to be pregnant] is it?... I'm not young and strong any more. There's no way I'd be able to raise it. So I went to Bangkok. My younger sister is in Bangkok so she took me... They injected some medicine in. Made my stomach hurt. I gave birth just the same as you'd give birth to a child. I didn't know how they did it, I just lay down. Lay down on a bed and gave birth there on the bed itself. I could see young people, they were crying, it wasn't just me who was there. They had nurses, but the doctors, they did their work. But they looked after me. Once they had gotten the *tua* [body] to come out, a *luuk* [child] came out, see. But it wasn't very big, quite small, just over two months. When it came out the pain went away just like giving birth to a child. They had me lie in the hospital for a night...

And Auntie when they injected you, did they give you saline?

They didn't inject me. They gave it [the medicine] to me by way of the *nam kleua* [saline intravenous drip]. Once the saline and the medicine had gone in I had stomach pain straight away. Then it was just one lump. It was just the same as giving birth to a child...

Did you lose a lot of blood?

No, no I didn't lose a lot, normal. I'd have to tell you straight that it was comfortable. But the young girls who went to do it, three months'

> [gestation], five months', dangerous. But the doctors took good care of them. But they were in a lot of pain. I saw kids, they'd be all bent up, *Wooh!* crying....

Aunty Phim is a rice farmer with four years of education and lives in a village in Roi Et province in northeast Thailand. She has two daughters. One daughter (twenty years old) is already married and the other (fourteen years old) is still in school. The abortion cost five thousand baht (approximately US$ 100), or two thousand baht per month of gestation – nearly a third of her yearly family income. Following the abortion she was given medicine to treat infection, vitamins and pain killers.

> *What sort of feelings do you have now that you have gone to do it?*
>
> I've been to do it. There. I feel that we won't have any obligation to feel anxious over that child. I won't have to think about lots of different things and try to be happy that I have to raise a child, anything like that. I'm old already. We could raise them but not well enough. Now the thinking has gone away, I don't have to think any more. I just think it was born just thus far and I'll let it go according to merit [the Buddhist understanding of the balance of good and bad deeds during one's life]. Some people, they say to correct it I should make merit.

Aunty Laem

Aunty Laem is thirty-six years old and married with two children, one son aged three and one daughter aged four. She has had four years of education. She is also a rice farmer with more debt than income. Last year she had an abortion when she was approximately three months' pregnant. She hadn't been using contraceptives. She went to a local woman's house who gave her an injection per vagina. The abortion cost her two thousand baht [US$ 40]:

> She put medicine into a syringe and injected it into my vagina. It was black medicine, black but not very strong so I had no problem and no symptoms, it was just normal. Then I returned home and on the second day it [the pregnancy] came out. It came out normally like I had my periods but the last lump was big – then I had cramps and didn't feel very good. When the last lump came out I was OK. She said what she would do for me and she said that if I died or anything she wouldn't take responsibility and I said that I needed it and accepted that. But lots of people go. Lots of people from our village and [they]

> don't have any problem... She said it was *bap* [Buddhist sin] but only a small sin and not really a problem...
>
> My child was still breastfeeding so I wasn't ready and so I decided... I spoke with my friends and I decided we lacked any other path. So I forced myself to do it. We weren't ready to have another child and so what can you do? We didn't have any money and so it was a necessity.

Following the abortion, Aunty Laem started using injectable contraception and now is using the contraceptive pill. She has had a number of women come to ask her about her experience of abortion and has referred them to the woman.

> Now I think about it and I am not happy. I'm scared I will catch something. I am scared it will become something like cancer. Scared I may have caught AIDS or something. Five people went to do it [abortions when she was there]. That's how I think in my heart. But before I went I didn't think about that... But I hope I didn't catch anything. But I saw lots of people being done. No one had anything.

Aunty Phim and Aunty Laem shared their stories with me in 1997 during fieldwork in Thailand. At that time Thailand had one of the most restrictive abortion laws in the region, allowing legal abortion only in the case of rape, incest and a threat to the health of the mother, which was usually interpreted very narrowly. Debate over Thailand's abortion laws has raged publicly since 1980, pitting Thai women's groups and public health advocates against popular conservative politicians, a Buddhist religious sect and a sensationalist media. In these debates, abortion became a metaphor for westernisation, changing gender roles, and political corruption – a threat to cherished notions of what it means to be Thai and to be a Buddhist (Whittaker 2004). Within that debate the experience of women was rarely voiced. Faced with their personal dilemmas of unplanned pregnancies and uncertain futures, women acted with pragmatism to address their situations. But their choices were structured within the broader political-economic and legal context. For Aunty Phim that involved a technically illegal abortion under medical supervision but in conditions that fell short of high-quality care. After unsuccessful attempts with 'hot women's medicines' (local herbal mixtures said to act as abortifacients), Aunty Laem resorted to the services of a local injection abortionist. Both women were aware of the illegality of their act and possible risks. They were fortunate they did not suffer adverse complications, although they knew women who had. Aunty Phim looks back with relief and few

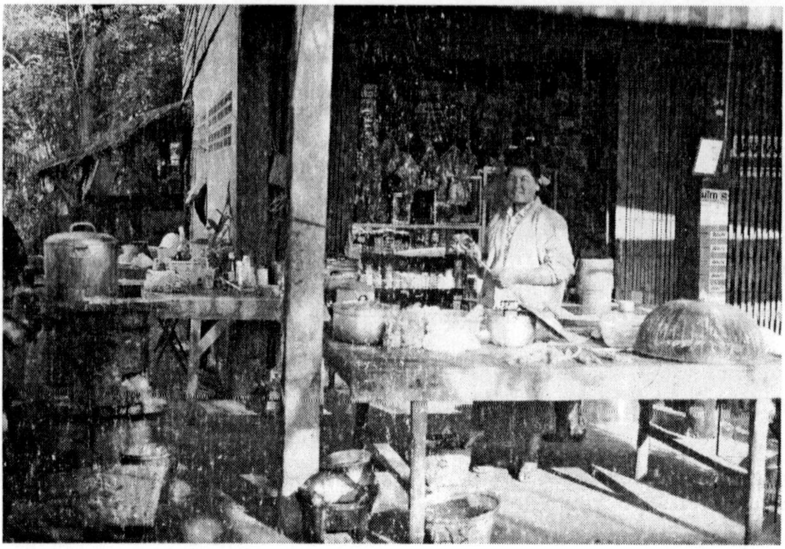

Illustration 1.1 Small village stores in Thailand often stock herbal medicines and other patent drugs purchased by women in attempts to induce abortions (Photograph: A. Whittaker)

regrets. Aunty Laem still worries about the unknown karmic consequences of her act but also fears long-term problems – AIDS from the use of shared equipment, or uterine cancer believed to derive from the disruption to the womb.

Raising the Issue

Writing about abortion forces us to confront the effects of poverty and economic inequalities, the configurations and expectations of gender relations, the meanings attributed to motherhood, the value of children, local moral worlds and understandings of women's bodies. The authors in this book articulate the conditions and hard choices faced by women throughout Asia. We relate stories of women's experiences with abortion as well as the politics surrounding abortion reforms. We describe how structural factors such as the distribution of economic, political and institutional resources are fundamental to the degree of control women and men have over reproductive decision-making and how cultural processes shape the contexts and meanings of their reproductive decisions. This draws attention to state interventions into their citizens' reproductive lives and the macro and micro relations of power, class and gender politics influencing reproductive experiences.

This book is also about the progress and possibilities for change. Despite the vociferous debate in Thailand, reform to the medical regulations governing abortion occurred in 2006 through the patient lobbying and quiet determination of a group of public health advocates and women's advocates working within existing bureaucratic and legal systems (see Nongluk Boonthai et al. this volume). This has made pregnancy terminations permissible under some circumstances such as for certain foetal conditions and mental health reasons, easing access to safe abortion services for some women. Despite this progress, abortion remains in the Thai Criminal Code and remains illegal for social and economic reasons as described by Aunty Phen and Aunty Laem. Work towards reform continues.

My ethnographic work in Thailand alerted me to the need for a volume bringing together current social research on abortion in Asia, in order to bring the diverse perspectives and insights from this region to a wider audience and to encourage further research of the consequences and implications of unsafe abortion in the region and the need for access to quality services. To date, relatively few books have addressed abortion in Asia.[1] This is surprising, given that the majority of the world's population lives in Asia and that over half of the world's deaths due to unsafe abortion take place in Asia.

This book aims to present a set of chapters detailing current work in Asia on abortion that reflect the diversity of experiences and perspectives from parts of the region usually under-represented in academic work, and to provide commentary on contemporary developments and understandings of the issue. The authors present cases ranging from nations with liberal abortion laws to those with strict restrictions, and highlight the fact that liberal laws alone do not ensure safe abortion services. Written by a mixture of Asian and Western researchers and activists, the book is comprised of eleven chapters that juxtapose anthropological descriptions of the lived experience of abortions with overviews of policy development and legal reform in the region. The contributors in this volume draw upon anthropology, demography, women's studies, public health and development studies in their approaches, and so the chapters require reading across disciplines but also across language written for different purposes. This book is intended to be a dialogue between academics and advocates and between anthropology and public health. The chapters are linked by their common attention to the cultural and historical specificities of abortion in each setting and their common underlying advocacy of the reproductive rights and entitlements of women and men to control their fertility.

The authors address a range of issues of importance in approaches to abortion, such as the difficulties faced by providers of reproductive health services to vulnerable populations; the linkages between violence and abortion; patients' assessment of quality of care versus costs of abortions; the sensitivity and care required of health providers for women experiencing mid-trimester or later term abortions for medical reasons; and the necessary collaboration with government ministries and other strategies employed for policy and legal reform. Through the use of anthropological methods, a number of authors are able to present insights into the micro-politics of gender relations and the lived experiences of abortion decision-making with a depth not possible through other, more quantitative means. The final chapters remind us of the dogged persistence and negotiations required to implement legal and policy reforms and the need to defend hard-won successes in reproductive rights. The book is ambitious in that it attempts to provide insights into the diversity of Asian countries, cultures, religions and historical experience. It will quickly become clear to readers that one cannot necessarily assume commonalities between 'Asian' countries and their approaches to the issue of abortion. As the essays in this book demonstrate, across the region different political systems, religious groups, colonial and postcolonial histories and legal developments have all influenced the nature of women's access to abortion.

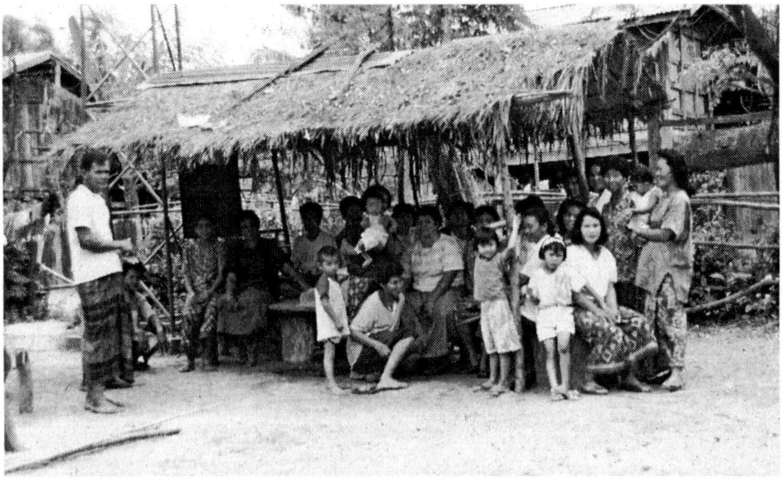

ILLUSTRATION 1.2 Northeast Thai village women gathered for a focus group (Photograph: A. Whittaker).

Counting the Costs

It has become a public health mantra to cite the International Conference on Population and Development (ICPD) 1994 statement that in circumstances where they are legal, abortions should be safe, and that all women should have access to life-saving post-abortion care (PAC) services. The Fourth World Conference on Women (FWCW) further called upon governments to consider reviewing laws containing punitive measures against women who have undergone illegal abortions (United Nations 1996, paragraph 106) and reaffirmed the human rights of women in the area of sexual and reproductive health, including their right to 'decide freely and responsibly the number, spacing and timing of their children and to have the information and means to do so, and their right to attain the highest standard of sexual and reproductive health' (United Nations 1995, paragraph 7.3). Despite much activity and rhetoric over reproductive health rights, over a decade later this commitment remains a distant goal for most countries in the Asian region.

The statistics speak for themselves. Approximately 10.5 million unsafe abortions take place in Asia each year, almost one for every seven live births. An unsafe abortion is one 'either by persons lacking the necessary skills or in an environment lacking the minimal medical standards, or both' (WHO 2003: 12). Thirty per cent of unsafe abortions in Asia are performed on women under twenty-five years of age and 60 per cent are obtained by women aged under thirty (Aahman and Shah 2004). It is estimated that each year 35,000 women in Asia lose their lives due to unsafe abortions, around half of the global deaths from unsafe abortion (Shah 2004). Apart from maternal death, at least one in five women suffer reproductive tract infections causing infertility as a result of their unsafe abortions (WHO 2003: 14). Complications from abortions are also costly to health services; it is estimated that in 2005, five million women across the world were admitted to hospitals due to complications caused by unsafe abortions (Singh 2006).

For many women in Asia, abortion and its consequences remain a common threat to their sexual and reproductive health. Many women do not yet have access to basic safe abortion services or post-abortion care. Instead, many women such as Aunty Phim and Aunty Laem face induced abortions in fear, pain and insecurity, seeking treatment wherever it is available, often at high cost to themselves and their families. 'Deciding freely' or 'choice' as it is articulated within the international human rights documents is bound up with

Western notions of the autonomous rational individual subject who rationally selects between the available options. As the chapters of this book reveal, the 'right to choose' is not a mere question of the legality of abortion, but depends upon questions of culture, political economy, class and gender relations.

Regional Overview

In almost all countries in Asia laws permit abortion to save a woman's life. However, considerable variation exists in the legal permissibility in other circumstances. Debates have taken place over the relationship between the legalisation of abortion and rates of maternal mortality. A study of 160 countries found that, in general, those with liberal abortion laws had a lower incidence of unsafe abortion and lower mortality from unsafe abortions when compared to those countries where abortion is restricted (Berer 2004). The countries with the most restricted abortion laws in Asia include Sri Lanka, Pakistan and the Philippines. Those with the least restrictions include Cambodia, Vietnam and China. It must be noted that this refers to the legality of abortion in various states' Criminal or Penal codes and may accurately reflect neither the 'grey law' regulatory frameworks which operate in various locations, nor the enforcement of that law. As will become evident below in the selected national profiles, a range of administrative and regulatory barriers restricting women's access to abortion services may operate even in states with liberal laws. The overview also illustrates that access to safe abortion services remains limited in most localities, whether because of economic or social barriers, the negative attitudes of health providers, or the failure of health systems to provide quality comprehensive reproductive health services. For example, in India, where abortion has been legalised for three decades, the high rate of unsafe abortion continues to be an issue (Ramachandar and Pelto 2002; Pallikadavath and Stones 2006). As the overview also reveals, there is a lack of comprehensive data on the prevalence of unsafe abortions. Legal restrictions make the collection of such data even more difficult and render the extent of unsafe abortions and the injuries to women invisible.

Unwanted pregnancies and the unsafe abortions which follow them are indicators of the gendered economic, social and political inequalities in societies and the extent to which women's needs and interests are not recognised or addressed. Trade liberalisation, structural adjustment programmes and the 1997 Asian economic crisis have negatively affected economic inequalities and the availability of national public resources for social programmes and public health interventions. Health care has become increasingly privatised across the region and less accessible to the poor. Economic barriers have limited both governments' abilities to implement quality reproductive health programmes of the sort recommended by the Cairo Population and Development Conference, as well as affecting individual women's access to quality services. In many countries in the region, risk of and from unsafe abortion is stratified along economic lines: regardless of the legal situation, the wealthy can access safe abortions, while the poor cannot.

It is impossible to separate discussion of abortion from the relations of power structuring gender relations and sexuality (Hardacre 1997). A pattern evident across the region is that strongly patriarchal societies tend to have a greater prevalence of unsafe and clandestine abortions. Persistent gender inequalities in education, marriage, citizenship, employment, property and political participation experienced by women affect their ability to control their fertility, negotiate their reproductive health needs with their families and health services, locate safe providers, mobilise money or influence political debate. In particular, poorer women in South Asian countries often have little control over decision-making within their families, with decisions over their fertility often being made by other family members. Likewise, women may have little ability to use contraceptives without their husband's permission and hence are at risk of unwanted pregnancies and subsequent abortions. Each chapter of the present volume engages in its own way with the politics of gender relations and societies' expectations of women and men. The meanings of abortion and the experiences of women undergoing abortion reveal much about the status of women in a society. The meanings of abortion vary in differing cultural systems where the social value of women depends upon their ability to bear children, or the number of children they bear, or the paternity of those children, or the sex of those children. As these chapters describe, in countries where abortion remains illegal, punitive measures almost invariably target women seeking abortions, not men. Transformations in gender relations wrought through social changes such as industrialisation, increased education for women, rural–urban migration and increased participation in the workforce, the effects of conflict, and state policies are all reflected in the practices and meanings of abortion and competing constructions of sexuality and motherhood.

Although Western scholars tend to emphasise religion in determining attitudes and practices regarding abortion, this is based on the assumption that religion carries the same influence in other countries as it does in determining practices, policies and debates in countries such as the United States. On the contrary, an analysis in the region reveals that countries with similar religious profiles may in fact carry very different legal approaches and different attitudes to the issue of abortion. For example, despite both having a majority Muslim population, Malaysia and Indonesia vary greatly in the restrictiveness of their abortion laws. Countries with Mahayana Buddhist traditions as practiced in Japan, Korea, China, Taiwan and Vietnam show greater tolerance for abortion than those with Theravada Buddhist traditions such as Thailand, Laos and Sri Lanka, yet Cambodia (also Theravada Buddhist) has very liberal laws. How can we account for such differences? A significant explanation can be found if we differentiate the particular religion practised from the degree to which a religion is associated with state legitimation. This varies from place to place, depending upon the colonial histories and legal structures inherited by states; the degree to which religion is mobilised as a unifying force in nationalist projects by the state; contemporary political histories, including the growth of politically active fundamentalist religious movements; and the involvement of the military in national politics. To put it simply, I suggest that it is when religion and nation become mutually supportive that we may expect the enforcement of restrictive abortion laws and intense sanctions against abortion.

As will be discussed later in this chapter, prospects for change in the region vary. The restriction or absence of civil society organisations or a strong established feminist movement affects the ways in which abortion reform advocates can mobilise support or educate the public about the effects of unsafe abortion, or counter gender stereotypes. In a number of countries, much progress has been made to reform laws and policies as part of the implementation of ICPD principles, and most importantly to improve the delivery of services. Yet in others, the growing political influence of religious fundamentalisms threaten to erode progress in the provision of a range of reproductive health services. The region has also been subject to international politics, affecting donor contributions to their reproductive health programmes, the ability of organisations to provide abortion services, to lobby for abortion rights, or to undertake programme research.

Finally, it is clear from the overview below that many countries in Asia continue to struggle to provide quality family planning services or appropriate post-abortion care, and lack staff trained in the safest techniques. In many cases this is due to governments assigning a low priority to funding for reproductive health. Paradoxically, while the agenda for reproductive health services has become more ambitious following ICPD and Beijing, it becomes so at a time of a parallel shifts in the national priorities of many countries and a withdrawal of the state from the provision of health services. When reproductive health services are left solely to private services, the potential for exploitation and high cost to clients increases. In addition, in poorly resourced public services, the quality of care received by patients can be very low (Ramachandar 2005). In those countries where abortion continues to be highly restricted, women and medical professionals may face fines and imprisonment. In these locations women often have few options but to seek the services of untrained practitioners utilising a range of techniques with little follow-up care. They may also fear presenting to medical services if complications occur.

The following profiles of a selection of countries in Asia briefly describes the current capacity of women to access safe abortion services in the country and serves as background to the following chapters. Not all countries are represented, nor is much information available on the situation in some countries such as North Korea or Bhutan. These profiles do serve, however, to highlight the diversity of approaches to the issue across the region.

Country Profiles

Southeast Asia

Thailand

As I have described in previous work (Whittaker 2004) the current criminal code and regulations in Thailand regarding abortion make it illegal except in cases of a women's health or in the case of rape or incest. Amendments to the medical regulations in 2006 made it possible for women to obtain abortions in the case of rape or foetal impairment, and the definition of health has been expanded to include the mental health of the woman as a factor in legal abortion provision (Royal Thai Government 2005), although no change to the Penal Code occurred. This will allow for increased access to abortion for some women. But access to pregnancy terminations will remain difficult for the majority of women who seek them on economic grounds, or for adolescents experiencing an unwanted pregnancy

(Warakamin et al. 2004), forcing them to resort to illegal means. My own work on abortion in Thailand described how Thai abortion laws operate to stratify the risk: poorer rural women or embarrassed, uninformed adolescents tend to seek unsafe illegal abortions, while richer, middle-class urban women can afford to have their illegal but safe abortions in private clinics and hospitals (Whittaker 2004). Despite the legal restrictions, approximately 300,000 abortions take place in Thailand each year. Research conducted in public hospitals in 1999 found that 32.1 per cent of women who presented to public hospitals following abortions suffered serious complications (Warakamin et al. 2004).

Public debates in Thailand over abortion legal reform throughout the 1980s and 1990s constructed abortion as un-Buddhist, anti-religious and therefore un-Thai behaviour (Whittaker 2004). Those opposing repeated attempts to reform abortion laws in the Thai parliament described abortion as the product of corrupt Western materialist values that threaten the integrity of the Thai nation and Thai values. A repeated theme throughout these debates was patriarchal concerns with women's body boundaries as icons of the borders of the nation within which Thai citizens are nurtured. Women seeking an abortion are depicted as having uncontrolled sexuality and Western proclivities; in their parallel role as 'mothers of the nation', they are also therefore depicted as threatening to destroy/abort the nation. Abortive technologies are thus positioned as instruments of evil, threatening the body of the nation and hence are strictly regulated.

Laos and Union of Myanmar (Burma)

Two other predominantly Buddhist nations have highly restrictive abortion laws. Little information is available about abortion in Laos; however, abortion is illegal except to save a woman's life (United Nations 2007a). Abortion is also illegal in Myanmar according to section 312A of the Penal Code, and strong social sanctions against abortion affect women's ability to seek care. With a low prevalence of contraception (estimated at only 34 per cent in urban areas and 10 per cent in rural areas), complications from induced abortions remain a major public health problem. This problem is particularly acute in conflict areas on Myanmar's borders and in rural areas with poor health services. Estimates of the incidence of women admitted for complications from abortion (both induced and spontaneous) vary, but are assumed to account for up to 60 per cent of direct obstetric deaths recorded in hospital-based studies (Ba-Thike 1997:

94). By 1995, abortion was ranked as the ninth most important health problem and ranked third among the leading causes of morbidity in Myanmar. Crude methods such as the insertion of abortion sticks or feathers, metal rods, or drugs into the uterus, curettage or external massage, as well as the consumption of herbal medicines are common methods used to induce abortions (Ba-Thike 1997; Belton 2001). Under the current regime, there has been little debate over the issue in Myanmar, although there are current efforts to introduce better protocols for the treatment of post-abortion complications within the health system (Htay et al. 2003). It is unclear what opposition groups' policies will be on this issue.

Cambodia

Despite having similar Theravada Buddhist traditions to those of Thailand and Laos, Cambodia has liberal abortion laws following legislation enacted in 1997 despite the opposition of some groups who argued that it was against Buddhist values. Abortion is available on request in the first twelve weeks of pregnancy but must be performed by medical doctors and medical assistants or by secondary midwives who are authorised to perform abortions. Abortion must be carried out in hospitals, health centres or clinics authorised by the Ministry of Health. After twelve weeks, abortion can be performed on the ground of foetal abnormality or if the pregnancy poses a danger to the mother's life; if the baby who will be born 'can get an incurable disease' (*sic*) or if the pregnancy is caused by rape. In such cases, the abortion requires the approval of a group of '2 or 3 medical personnel' (United Nations 2007b).

Cambodia's legislation was adopted in an attempt to reduce the country's high maternal mortality rate of 900 per 100,000 live births, of which it was estimated that one third of maternal mortality resulted from unsafe abortions performed by unskilled practitioners. According to the 2000 Demographic and Health Survey, 6 per cent of women aged fifteen to forty-nine reported at least one previous abortion. Primarily the difficulty is the impoverished health system. Cambodia is one of the poorest countries in the Asian region, struggling to provide services to its population after years of conflict. There is little access to quality family planning services in the country and this is combined with widespread fear of contraceptive side effects, resulting in many unplanned pregnancies (Sadana and Snow 1999). Few government clinics have the training or personnel to offer abortion services, so women must travel to the capital, Phnom Penh, for services. Reports suggest that few people are even aware that abortion services are legal and available to women, and there is widespread self-medication using drugs purchased over the counter (including substances such as strychnine) as well as the continued use of traditional techniques such as massage and the insertion of objects for the induction of abortions. A study of sex workers in Cambodia found that abortion was widely utilised due to low contraceptive use, but that it was perceived to be risky and costly (Deavaux et al. 2003).

Vietnam

Apart from Cambodia, Vietnam has the most liberal abortion laws. The 1989 Law on Protection of People's Health recognises a woman's right to decide to have an abortion. Vietnamese women have one of the highest rates of abortion in the world, estimated at 2.5 abortions per woman during her lifetime (Henshaw et al. 1999). A major goal of the National Reproductive Health Care Strategy 2001–2010 in Vietnam is to reduce the number of unwanted pregnancies and to manage abortion-related complications effectively (Centre for Reproductive Rights and ARROW 2005: 219). Vietnam's abortion rate reflects a history of poor quality of care and lack of choice within family planning services throughout Vietnam along with a lack of post-abortion contraceptive counselling. The use of mifepristone and misoprostol for medical abortion was introduced into the Vietnam National Reproductive Health Guidelines in 2002 (Ganatra et al. 2004) and is now available as a choice in public clinics for early terminations alongside MVA. Sex-selective abortions were banned by the government in 2006 (see the chapter by Wolf et al., this volume).

Philippines

In the Philippines, the strong influence of the Catholic Church sustains highly restrictive abortion legislation which only allows abortion to save the life of a woman. The Philippines 1987 constitution defines human life as existing from conception and grants the foetus equal rights with a pregnant woman: '[the state] shall equally protect the life of the mother and the life of the unborn from conception'. The Revised Penal Code (1930) imposes a range of penalties for women undergoing abortion, including imprisonment. Similarly, health professionals providing abortion services may have their licenses to practice revoked. Despite the restrictions, it is estimated that 400,000 unsafe abortions occur each year in the Philippines (Centre for Reproductive Rights and ARROW 2005: 139), most obtained through traditional birth attendants, midwives and doctors acting illegally (Cadelina 1999). The abortion issue remains a highly emotive one, in which the Catholic Church maintains a vociferous campaign against any reproductive health reforms, including discouraging the use of contraceptives. The Catholic campaign is supported by a worldwide Catholic network and uses a range of tactics and organisations, including sophisticated marketing campaigns utilising foetocentric imagery to mobilise moral outrage; targeted political efforts to support and elect members of parliament to help prevent the passage of legislative reform bills; and the support of Catholic medical associations to impact on health professionals' willingness to provide appropriate care. Women's groups are depicted in these campaigns as anti-family and immoral. In 2001, the emergency contraceptive Postinor was banned on the grounds that it was considered an abortifacient; however, a review of that decision has since determined that it is both legal and safe (Centre for Reproductive Rights and ARROW 2005: 139).

Indonesia and Malaysia

Malaysia and Indonesia form an interesting comparison. Both nations have a majority Muslim population, both inherited restrictive colonial legal legacies, and both share emerging fundamentalist religious movements that are increasingly politically influential. As Hull and Widyantoro note in this book, Indonesia has a number of laws governing the provision of abortion: under Articles 346–348 of the Penal Code, all abortions are prohibited. However, article 15 of the Law on Health gives an exception to this law, allowing 'certain medical actions' to be performed to save the life of 'the pregnant mother and/or her foetus'. Despite the efforts of women's organisations, the growing strength and influence of fundamentalist Islamic political parties makes the prospect for legal reforms unlikely in the near future and indeed threatens a range of reproductive health services.

By contrast, Malaysia has a liberal abortion law, yet it suffers from a lack of implementation (see Rashidah Abdullah and Yut-Lin Wong, this volume). Health providers are reluctant to provide abortion services, even to women who are legally entitled to services, and there is widespread misunderstanding and confusion about the legal provisions governing abortion. Although there has been agreement between Islamic leaders over the permissibility of abortion under certain conditions, there is a widespread misconception that abortion is totally forbidden under Islam. Nine abortion-related deaths were reported in Malaysia in 2002 (Centre for Reproductive Rights and ARROW 2005: 18, 96).

Timor-Leste

Timor-Leste experiences high maternal death and fertility rates. Sources suggest a maternal mortality rate of 800/100,000 to 890/100,000, or double that of Indonesia (Povey and Mercer 2002; UNDP 2006). The accuracy of this figure is doubtful given the lack of reliable statistical data in Timor-Leste. It is likely, however, that complications from unsafe abortions contribute to a high maternal mortality. rate. Although the exact number of induced abortions currently taking place in Timor-Leste is unknown, evidence from three of its four hospitals suggest that 40 per cent of all emergency obstetric care involves managing and treating complications from early pregnancy losses. Post-abortion care in hospitals remains limited and does not utilise evidence based protocols. Access to family planning information, education and supplies is limited especially for vulnerable groups such as young people (Belton, Whittaker and Barclay 2009).

In 2005, East Timorese lawmakers began drafting a Penal Code for the new nation, an opportunity to revise the highly restrictive Indonesian laws left over from Indonesian occupation, which currently makes abortion illegal in all cases, even when a woman's life is in danger. Debate and consultation on this continues, with women's organisations, other NGO representatives, members of the Catholic Clergy, officials of the Ministry of Health and the UN Specialised Agencies participating in public fora on the issue. The National Reproductive Health Strategy of the government of Timor-Leste supports the provision of modern methods of contraception and access to post-abortion care, although is not supportive of access to abortion services. The influence of the Catholic Church remains strong and affects attitudes towards the provision and use of contraception and abortion.

East Asia

China

China's notorious one-child policy has produced a range of human rights abuses, including forced abortions (for discussion see Greenhalgh and Winkler 2005; Greenhalgh 2003). The Chinese policies generated enormous controversy in the West and influenced political decisions in the U.S. and Australia to restrict donor funding to organisations working in China. Although in recent years the one-child policy has been relaxed and greater emphasis has been placed upon improving the quality of the family planning programme, concerns remain about the quality of care, especially pain control and health consequences for women undergoing abortions (Zhou Weijin et al. 1999). Abortion is available on request up to six months' gestation, with the consent of family and spouse. Despite an extensive family planning programme, in 1999 four million abortions took place in China, but reliable statistics are difficult to locate (Centre for Reproductive Rights 2005: 45–46). Non-medical sex-selective abortions are strictly prohibited by the Population and Family Planning Law (2002) (Centre for Reproductive Rights and ARROW 2005: 45), yet despite this prohibition, the practice is known to continue (Chu Junhong 2001; Löfstedt et al. 2004).

Taiwan

Abortion was legalised in Taiwan in 1985, although before that time, abortion was readily available. By the 1990s nearly one third of all pregnancies were terminated. As Moskowitz (2001) notes, abortion is common in Taiwan, yet it is also seen as an act which defies Confucian ideals of filial responsibility to continue the family line, Buddhist beliefs regarding the sinfulness of killing sentient life, and challenges dominant Taiwanese cultural ideals of women as nurturers. As in Japan, temples and religious masters across Taiwan offer appeasement services for foetus ghosts, sometimes at considerable cost (see discussion of similar understandings in Vietnam from Gammeltoft, this volume).

Japan

Japan is notable for its ready social acceptance of abortion. Its abortion rate is among the highest in the world, with an estimated two-thirds of Japanese women having had an abortion by age forty (Oaks 1994). This is partly due to the fact that, until recently, government restrictions have limited the availability of the contraceptive pill on 'public hygiene grounds'. It has been argued that the continued limits placed on oral contraceptives has also ensured the continuation of a lucrative abortion business by physicians.

Under the Eugenics Protection Law of 1948, abortion on demand is legal in Japan up to twenty-two weeks' gestation if a 'woman's health may be affected seriously by continuation of pregnancy or childbirth from the physical or economic viewpoint' (Oaks 1994: 513). The Eugenics Protection Law was reformed during the post-war occupation of Japan. The clause allowing abortions to be performed in cases of economic hardship was included in 1949 and in 1952, restrictions requiring that each case be approved by a local eugenics council were abolished, allowing individual physicians to judge their patients' needs (Hardacre 1997: 56–57).

As Hardacre notes, challenges to the Eugenics Protection Law in Japan have come from the 'new' religion *Seicho no Ie* which especially focuses on the soul and views abortion as homicide. In 1964, it founded a conservative right-wing nationalist political lobbying group called the *Seicho no Ie Seiji Rengo* (The Political Association of *Seicho no Ie*). A number of attempts have been made to restrict the law in Japan, spearheaded by *Seicho no Ie* with support from Japanese Catholic groups. The campaign to change the Eugenics bill reached its zenith in the early 1980s (coinciding with a similar campaign in Thailand) when a fifth and final campaign failed in 1983. Opposition to the *Seicho no Ie* campaign by Japanese feminists mobilised a coalition of doctors and family planners in opposition to the move to eliminate the economic hardship condition in the law (Hardacre 1997: 76–77). Although small campaigns to oppose abortion continue to be active during provincial elections, these have not attracted widespread support.

South Korea

South Korea makes an interesting contrast to Japan in that it shares liberal attitudes towards abortion. However, abortion remains technically illegal except in limited circumstances. Attempts to liberalise the law in 1966 and 1970 failed. A Maternal and Child Health Law was passed in 1973 by a martial law authority permitting abortions with the consent of a woman and her spouse in cases of hereditary defects in the foetus, certain infectious diseases, when a pregnancy resulted from rape or incest, or when the pregnancy is deemed to be detrimental to the health of the mother. However, despite the technical ban on abortions, the laws are not enforced. Korean society in general is very tolerant of abortion and obtaining one is relatively easy. Common estimates posit that approximately one million abortions are induced annually (Tedesco 1999: 130). Due to a strong son preference, sex-selective abortions are common and are resulting in a distorted gender ratio in the country, despite the fact that legislation passed in 1987 and 1994 made prenatal sex selection illegal. Tedesco notes that Buddhist groups in Korea have generally not been involved in the abortion issue, with the Catholic Church instead leading opposition to liberalisation.

South Asia

South Asia accounts for one third of the world's unsafe abortions. Unsafe abortion is a leading cause of death among women in South Asia: an estimated 29,000 women die every year in the region from unsafe abortion (Center for Reproductive Rights and ARROW 2005: 16). These figures reflect the generally low status of women and the gender inequalities in the region. However, they are also indicative of poverty, lack of access to health services, particularly family planning services, and restrictive legal frameworks in a number of countries.

Sri Lanka

Sri Lanka has a highly restrictive law regarding abortion dating from 1883, prohibiting abortion except when performed to save a woman's life. There is no national-level data on the incidence of abortion. However, it is estimated that around 25,000 to 30,000 abortions are induced each year. Abortion remains a leading cause of maternal death (Hewage 1999). A number of attempts have been made to reform the Sri Lankan Penal Code in order to relax restrictions on abortion. The most recent of these took place in 1995, when changes were proposed to parliament as part of a Penal Code Bill encompassing a number of women's issues to allow abortion in cases of rape or incest or in cases of foetal abnormality. As in Thai debates on the issue, arguments based upon notions of culture, religion or tradition were used to oppose any form of liberalisation and the clause liberalising abortion was deleted from the second reading of the Bill to parliament (Abeyesekera 1997). In addition, the civil war in Sri Lanka has also been used to justify the need for a pronatalist policy. Hence, abortion remains a criminal offence and women continue to be prosecuted by police.

India

According to government data, an estimated 1.7 per cent of pregnancies in India end in induced abortion; between four million and six million abortions are performed illegally, and unsafe abortion accounts for upwards of 9 to 16 per cent of maternal deaths (Center for Reproductive Rights and ARROW 2005). A study conducted in rural Southern India (Varkey et al. 2000) found that 65 per cent of abortions had been carried out by untrained practitioners, although there are indications that such a pattern may be changing (see Ramachandar and Pelto 2004). The 1971 Medical Termination of Pregnancy Act in India includes a range of indictors for safe abortions, including to save a woman's life or health or in cases of rape, contraceptive failure in married women, foetal abnormality or socio-economic hardship. Despite these liberal conditions, studies show that illegal abortions outnumber legal procedures. However, this does not mean that all illegal procedures are unsafe. On the contrary, a number of studies (Duggal and Ramachandran 2004; Ramachandar and Pelto 2004) demonstrated that in many cases, women chose to attend 'illegal' but medically trained providers who lacked the government registration to provide abortion care, because these providers' quality of care and outcomes were better than the government registered providers. Recent simplification of the regulations governing the type of clinic able to perform early abortions, as well as improvements in services at public clinics, is meant to address this problem (see the chapter by Ramachandar and Pelto, this volume).

Access and the quality of care in public-sector abortion services in India remain patchy. Inappropriate technologies, poor quality services and judgmental staff can lead women to choose more expensive private clinics. For the poorest women, cost may remain a barrier and hidden costs at public clinics may encourage them to seek unsafe abortions with unskilled providers. Likewise, unmarried women in particular still face difficulty accessing legal procedures and often seek unsafe abortions (Ganatra and Hirve 2002). Medication abortion is available in government-approved hospitals and at all registered abortion clinics and its use has become widespread, even in rural areas; however, ethnographic studies demonstrate considerable variability in its use among providers, with incorrect regimes and over-the-counter sales (Ramachandar and Pelto 2005).

The Pre Natal Diagnostic Techniques Act of 1994 prohibits sex determination of a foetus or informing a couple about the sex of their foetus. However, the ready accessibility of ultrasonography and other technologies to determine the sex of a foetus make the Act difficult to enforce and ensure a continuation of the strong preference for male children (George 2002; Nidadavolu and Bracken 2006). Studies also suggest an increase in sex-selective abortions. The sex ratio among children aged 0–6 declined steadily over the 1990s, from 945 girls per one thousand boys in 1991 to 927 girls per one thousand boys in 2001 (Center for Reproductive Rights and ARROW 2004: 17).

Research in India also raises questions about the presumed association between legal abortion and the enjoyment of reproductive and sexual rights. Studies indicate that the utilisation of induced abortions rather than of reversible contraceptives among married women in India is partly due to the lack of women's sexual and reproductive rights within marriage. Ravindran et al. (2004) found that non-consensual sex, sexual violence and women's inability to refuse their husbands' sexual demands appear to underlie the need for abortion in both younger and older women. A large number of women in that study were denied their sexual rights but were permitted, even forced, to terminate their pregnancies for reasons unrelated to their right to choose abortion. The relationship between violence, denial of sexual rights and abortion requires further investigation across Asia. Similarly, a study by Gupte et al. (1997) in rural Maharashta found that many women felt uneasy about abortion, but often found themselves in 'no choice' situations due to pressure from their husbands or family to undergo abortion, including sex-selective abortions. Most women were dissatisfied with the quality of services provided. Many used abortion as their means of fertility control due to their husband's lack of permission to use contraceptives.

Bangladesh

Abortion is illegal in Bangladesh under the penal code, except to save the life of the mother. In these cases abortion must be performed by a qualified physician in a hospital. However, official government policy allows menstrual regulation (MR) as a means of establishing non-pregnancy, as opposed to terminating a pregnancy. It is allowed up to eight weeks from the last menstrual period by a trained family welfare visitor under the supervision of a physician, and up to the tenth week by a licensed medical practitioner and is available for married women only. However, the term MR is commonly used to describe a range of procedures (see the chapter by Rashid in this volume). MR has been available in government health facilities since 1979 and a range of private clinics also provide MR and abortion services (Caldwell 1999). However, the quality of care remains poor (Chowdhury and Moni 2004). A study of 143 women who had had MR procedures in rural Bangladesh found that a quarter of the abortion procedures were dangerous or inadequate, and that the number of women who developed complications was very high (43 per cent); one death was reported (Ahmed et al. 1999).

Given the high number of clandestine abortions, figures estimating the prevalence of induced abortion in Bangladesh are likely to be underestimates. A total of 28,000 women die each year due to pregnancy-related causes, of which 8,000 deaths are estimated to be from abortion-related complications. Overall, about 26 per cent of all pregnancy-related deaths in Bangladesh are thought to be due to induced abortion, with one study suggesting that as many as 50 per cent of admissions to obstetric wards are for abortion-related complications (see Ahmed et al. 1999).

Nepal

Until 2002, Nepal had one of the most restrictive and punitive abortion laws in the region, which saw women jailed for between three and twenty years for having abortions (Ramaseshan 1997). According to a number of studies throughout the 1990s, over 54 per cent of all hospital admissions were for women with post-abortion complications. Unsafe abortion contributed significantly to the very high maternal mortality rate in Nepal (Tamang and Tamang 2005). One study found that unplanned pregnancy accounted for 95 per cent of induced abortion among women and that the majority of the women were not using contraceptives (Tamang et al.1999). Following a concerted public campaign by activists, Nepal reformed its abortion laws in 2002 to allow for the performance of abortions on request for women during the first trimester, and in the case of rape or incest, up to eighteen weeks' gestation. Abortions may also be performed at any time during pregnancy with the approval of a physician, if the pregnancy poses a danger for the life of the pregnant woman, her physical or mental health or in the case of disability in the foetus. The new law also prohibits the use of amniocentesis for the purposes of sex-selective abortions (Shakya et al. 2004; Thapa 2004). The Nepalese health system now faces the challenge to appropriately implement this legal change and to ensure access to abortion, particularly for rural women. Women continue to utilise local untrained practitioners or self-medicate with a range of allopathic and indigenous medicines available on the Nepalese market to induce abortions (Tamang and Tamang 2005). Likewise, a significant challenge exists in improving access to contraceptives, particularly among impoverished rural populations, as it is estimated that only 59 per cent of demand is currently being met (Shakya et al. 2004: 77).

Pakistan

Abortion is illegal in Pakistan unless the procedure is necessary to save the woman's life or to provide 'necessary treatment' under the Islamic Qisas and Diyat Ordinance (1990). Without policies defining the requirements for obtaining an abortion under the 'life' or 'necessary treatment' exceptions, the discretion to perform abortions rests with physicians, most of whom are reluctant to interpret the law liberally due to the risk of prosecution (Center for Reproductive Rights 2004: 170–171). Few government facilities provide abortion services even under those exceptions, and there is little data available on the incidence of abortion. Due to the highly restrictive laws on abortion, the majority of abortions are either self-induced or performed in clandestine clinics in urban areas, whereas in rural areas, they are performed by untrained practitioners. Mifepristone and misoprostol are available by prescription in Pakistan, although not for use as abortifacients (Center for Reproductive Rights 2004: 170–171).

Reproductive Rights and Abortion Reform: The Challenge for Activists

The synopses above reveal that across the region, there remain considerable gaps between law, practice and ideology. In many cases, the laws regulating abortion bear little relation to the realities of practice and become political weapons rather than protections for citizens (see Hull and Widyantoro, this volume). Religious values antithetical to abortion may bolster support for maintaining restrictive laws, but may not reflect the pragmatic actions of women when faced with unplanned pregnancies. Likewise, rhetoric claiming the implementation of the ICPD goals by governments may not be borne out when women seek to access services on the ground. Activists face challenges in bridging these gaps; in confronting the disparities between states' imaginaries and lived realities.

Across Asia, the notion of reproductive rights remains novel outside academic, NGO and policy circles. The very terms of reproductive rights discourse often do not translate easily into local languages. Petchesky (1998: 2) notes that the philosophical bases of principles of reproductive freedom rest in Western traditions, particularly the liberal notion of 'property in one's own person', which is not necessarily universal in Asian societies. This point forms the basis of critiques of the notion of reproductive rights from third world feminists. For example, Correa (1994: 77) argues that the emphasis on individual autonomy assumed in reproductive rights discourse is founded on the Western bourgeois concept of a discrete 'self', a concept that is inappropriate for many cultural settings in Asia. She suggests that the notion of bodily integrity be understood in the context of significant family, cultural, social and economic relationships and that rights discourses need to take account of collective identities (1994: 79). Likewise, the International Reproductive Rights Research Action Group (IRRRAG) adopted the term 'sense of entitlement' to capture their informants' negotiated subjective component of rights. It is based upon a notion of 'the self both as individual and constructed through ongoing interaction and interdependency with others' (Petchesky 1998: 12–13). Wolf et al. (this volume) argue for a position that recognises the cultural diversity in constructions of rights, including reproductive rights. For example, they suggest that the language of rights in Vietnam is frequently couched in terms of the good of society and the nation. The challenge, they suggest, is to respect and recognise differing approaches to rights discourses so that in practice the exercise of an individual's rights coincides with that of the broader social good. However, Correa (1994: 82) also offers an overarching principle: 'when cultural practices only consolidate women's subordination and damage women's physical integrity or their freedom to make decisions about their own lives, we must question them'.

Women's advocacy strategies for abortion rights have developed around two major approaches: the 'health rationale', framing abortion as a major contributing factor in women's mortality around the world, and the 'rights rationale', asserting that the right to terminate a pregnancy is one protected by fundamental principles of human rights (Correa 1994: 70–71). These principles are not mutually exclusive, however. Until recently, the 'health rationale' rather than the 'rights rationale' has been emphasised in advocacy work across Asia, stressing morbidity and mortality rates attributed to unsafe abortion and the economic costs to public health systems of treating complications from unsafe induced abortions. As Correa notes, the danger of this rationale is that the issue of abortion becomes seen as a technical medical problem placed in the hands of the medical profession, rather than as an issue that must recognise women's rights and place women's desires and expectations at the forefront of the debate. Read against each other, the final two chapters on Malaysia and Thailand in this volume illustrate this tension between medically directed reforms versus the need to assert the primacy of reproductive rights as the fundamental principle driving abortion reform. The emergence of a number of reproductive rights coalitions such as the Reproductive Rights Advocacy Alliance Malaysia (RRAAM), Women's Health Foundation (WHF) in Indonesia and the Women's Health and Reproductive Rights Foundation of Thailand

(WHRRF) mark a shift in emphasis towards a rights-based approach. Hessini (2005) calls for a synthesis between the public health and human rights approaches and strategic alliances between such organisations and other social movements working in social justice as a foundation for legal reforms.

Given the political realities and the lack of a strong women's movement in many nations, it is often necessary for reproductive rights advocates to find a 'middle path' towards change, undertaking the transformation of law and social policy in pragmatic, slow and incremental steps. While public campaigns have succeeded in some countries such as Nepal (Thapa 2004), reform movements in Asia more commonly involve very small numbers of committed people, gradually raising the profile of the issue in public, in policy circles and within health programmes. Well-designed research can play an important role in this process by supporting efforts towards reform.

However, debate on the issue of abortion and reproductive rights faces concerted opposition in many locations. As noted in the regional overview, conservative religious movements and their political allies often target the issue of abortion. I have previously documented the rise of the Buddhist Santi Asoke sect, which greatly influenced attempts to introduce abortion law reforms in Thailand throughout the 1980s (Whittaker 2004). Such campaigns often take on nationalist overtones, with reproduction linked to fears about the moral corruption of the nation-state and the protection of 'Asian values'. While depicting themselves as representing authentic local cultural, religious and national values in opposition to Western values, the campaigns of such groups often draw support from international 'pro-life' and Catholic organisations.

But it is not only local conservatives influencing abortion access and debate in the region. The restrictive U.S. government policies reinstated under the Bush presidency in January 2001, known as the Global Gag Rule, forbade the use of U.S. family planning funds by organisations that perform, advocate for, or provide medical referrals or counselling for abortion, even when those activities were supported by their own non-U.S. funds and were lawful under their own national legislation. The impact of these policies cannot be overstated. The U.S. Agency for International Development (USAID) is the biggest bilateral donor in the field of family planning and reproductive health. In this way, internal U.S. policy influenced and limited what governments and NGOs in Asia could undertake with both their own and donor money, thereby silencing debate, restricting public education and leading to vital projects losing their funding, even in countries where abortion is legal (Global Gag Rule Impact Project 2003; Crane and Dusenberry 2004). However, on 23 January 2009, the Obama administration lifted the ban, restoring funding to the United Nations Population Fund. While not directly funding abortion services, this will allow funding to resume to groups and NGOs that provide other services, including counseling about abortions. Likewise, in April 2009, the Australian government amended the AusAID Family planning guidelines which similarly restricted Australian aid funding to any services, education, training or information in regard to safe or unsafe abortion services for the past thirteen years. This illustrates how the internal politics of abortion in countries such as the U.S. or Australia have international ramifications with direct consequences for women in the region. It reminds us how funding and support for abortion as an issue of health and rights is especially vulnerable to international political trends.

Overview of the Book

Abortion in Asia begins with the personal stories of women and the factors influencing their need for induced abortion, their ability to access services and their experience of services. As Petchesky writes in her introduction to *Negotiating Reproductive Rights,* 'we need to situate ... [the concept of reproductive rights] within direct testimonies about the daily constraints and relationships through which women – across a variety of countries and cultures – engage in reproductive and sexual transactions' (1998: 1). A number of chapters written by anthropologists in this volume take up that challenge, offering poignant descriptions and first-hand accounts of women's lives and decision-making and placing these accounts at the centre of their analysis. It starts with an account of decision-making around contraception and the resort to crude abortion methods in Cambodia. It moves to an emotive account of late therapeutic terminations in Vietnam, drawing attention to the ambivalence, sense of loss, grief and ethical subjectivity such decisions involve. The book then moves to accounts exploring the broader structural issues and institutional violence impinging upon women's decisions on the Burmese border Burma and in Bangladeshi slums. In these chapters women are marginal to the health system and must act outside it. Women's considerations and negotiations with health systems are further highlighted in a chapter considering women's decisions around quality of care and cost. The final chapters offer views on changing health and legal systems through public health interventions and activism. In doing so, the book moves from the personal to the public: from the pragmatic actions of individuals to public activism, from acting outside and within health systems to changing them, from the micro-politics to macro-politics of reproduction.

Chapter Two explores women's decision-making with regard to family planning and the experience of unplanned pregnancy in Cambodia. The account of Oung's case highlights the cultural logic behind women's choice of use of contraceptives and the poor counselling and care received from local health services, which, in Oung's case, ultimately resulted in an unplanned pregnancy and unsafe termination. As the authors argue, despite Cambodia's liberal abortion laws, the legal status of abortion remains little understood in the country by both women and health professionals. Access to safe abortion services remains poor. Instead, women rely on the services of local women skilled in crude abortion techniques and self-care for any ensuing complications, with the attendant risks that this carries.

The tensions around religious beliefs and the act of abortion come into stark relief in a number of chapters. In my own work in northeast Thailand, I heard women speak of the private rituals they undertook both to seek protection before their abortions and to obtain reconciliation with the spirit of the foetus in order to ensure its reincarnation and to recognise one's responsibility in the act of terminating one's pregnancy. In Theravadhan Buddhist Thailand, public temple rituals like those common in Mahayana Buddhist countries such as Japan, Taiwan or Korea, which seek to placate the spirits of aborted foetuses, are not practiced. Instead, women struggle to find their own language and means of reconciling their acts with their beliefs. Similarly, in Chapter Three, Gammeltoft offers an empathetic exploration of the experiences and dilemmas posed for women aborting wanted pregnancies for medical reasons following ultrasonography. The dilemmas faced by women over whether to bury the foetus, and thereby recognise it as one does other family members who have died, entails not only religious beliefs but, as she notes, Vietnamese ways of grieving and coping with painful events and contested views over the pain of memories. Vietnamese women's decisions over these matters are not individual decisions but usually entail the advice and counsel of elders and involve relationships with the living as much as with the dead.

Gammeltoft's chapter demonstrates the power of detailed ethnography to allow us to enter into another person's experience. Through women's eyes, we starkly experience the insensitivity of health care providers, the unintentional cruelties and ignominious suffering caused by a lack of counselling and support. The reader is forced to confront and interrogate his or her cultural assumptions regarding the social status of a foetus and rituals surrounding death. In the ethnographic chapters in particular, a picture emerges of women submitting themselves for medical procedures surrounded by fear, a lack of information, misunderstandings, uncertainties and little support.

Chapter Four offers first-hand accounts of women's decision-making on the Thai-Myanmar border. Belton describes the daily realities of poverty, harassment by border patrols, domestic violence and suffering experienced by Burmese forced migrants, all forms of structural violence perpetuated against women in this region. Burmese migrant workers lose their jobs in Thailand if they fall pregnant, forcing many to procure abortions rather than face economic insecurity. The embodied symptom of 'weakness' becomes the language through which to express vulnerability. Poor post-abortion care, a lack of contraceptive counselling and the illegality of abortion contribute to the continuation of this cycle. The inadequacies of post-abortion care for women is a repeated theme throughout this book. Rather than finding quality care, support and counselling, women face inadequate care with outdated techniques, discrimination, little privacy, blame and in some cases forced sterilisation.

Several chapters in this book describe the ambiguous terms used by women to describe the act of abortion. These terms can refer to local ethno-gynaecological understandings of the processes of reproductive bodies and pregnancy, but they also index the moral frameworks informing women's actions. Descriptions of abortion as a prophylactic act of washing out the uterus, 'sweeping clean' the uterus through D&C (dilation and curettage), removal of a mere 'lump of blood', restoring blocked menstruation through MR, or tests to check for possible pregnancy are common across Asia. The use of ambiguous terms enables a conceptual space in which the act of abortion can be more easily accepted. Similarly, we find common humoral understandings of the process of pregnancy and the widespread use of self-administered 'hot' medicines as abortifacients and menstrual regulators; such patent 'women's medicines' are exported and marketed across the Asian region. Even modern pharmaceuticals considered 'hot' and other 'hot' substances such as aspirin and whiskey are consumed in the attempt to effect an abortion. Alongside the consumption of herbal preparations, the chapters also detail some of the more dangerous abortion techniques used, such as the insertion of sticks, leaf stems and feathers or the use of uterine mas-

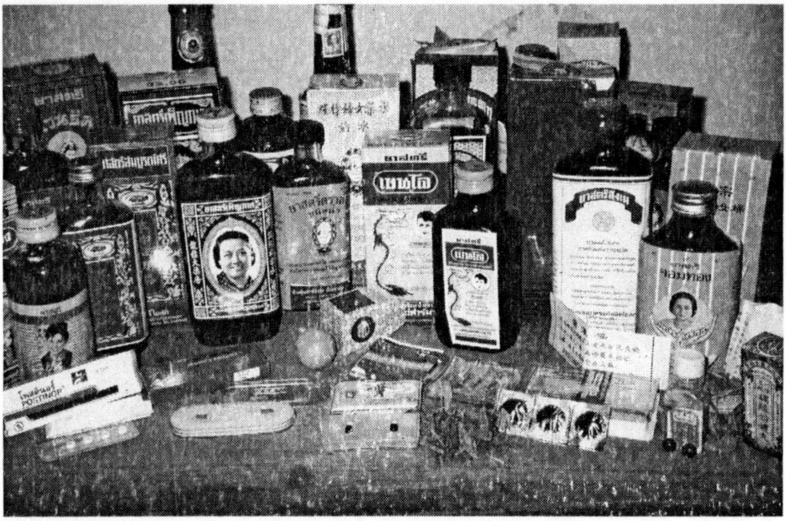

ILLUSTRATION 1.3 'Hot' medicines, herbal abortifacients and assorted contraceptives purchased over the counter from village stores in northeast Thailand, 1997 (Photograph: A. Whittaker).

sage or forceful pummelling. As a number of authors assert, local knowledge and availability of such techniques remains widespread, evidence of both the long history of abortion as a form of fertility control in the region and also of the continued dependence upon such techniques for many women. While many such abortions take place without complications, other women do experience complications and end up in the emergency departments of local hospitals.

The following chapter by Rashid gives married adolescent women's first-hand accounts of their reasons for abortion and experience of discrimination at the hands of health providers. Like the women described in Belton's chapter, these young woman are subject to personal and institutional violence and have little choice in the services they must use. Rashid's chapter speaks of the vulnerability of married adolescent women in Dhaka's slums, and how their poverty forces women to abort pregnancies and also determines the quality of care they receive. Poorly paid NGO health workers accompany women to private abortion providers rather than their own public health services in order to receive a small commission for each new client. The cry of frustration Rashid recalls from a woman left waiting to see a health worker, resonates for women around the world with regard to access to quality, safe abortion services: 'How long can we wait like this?'

In Chapter Six, Ramachandar and Pelto describe the costs involved in women's abortion-seeking in Tamil Nadu. They have worked for many years, collecting detailed observations of women's decision-making processes and the changes across time that have affected women's choices, including service provider attitudes and their ability to provide quality care. Due to a long-standing distrust in the quality of care at government clinics, poorer women will go into debt to pay for their abortions with providers that they consider offer good-quality care. But on a positive note, the up-grading of services in government primary health clinics (PHC) over the last few years has yielded improvements in the quality of services compared to what they observed in their previous work (Ramachandar, 2004 a,b). This also appears to have contributed to a decrease in the proportion of women they find seeking unqualified providers.

A further theme developed in this book is that of advocacy and the strategies used in the region to reform laws and assert the importance of women's reproductive rights at the national level. Chapter Seven provides a perspective from international NGO workers on collaboration with the Vietnamese government to improve service delivery and quality of care and to integrate principles of reproductive rights into government programmes. This chapter places abortion in a broader social and political context and gives an insight into the language used within policy changes. It also documents the Vietnamese government's attempts to both expand contraceptive availability and use and to improve abortion services in response to the high demand for abortion. The authors note the impact that U.S. policies such as the Global Gag Rule have had on donor funding for abortion programme work in Vietnam. They also make the observation that the sudden availability of large funds for other reproductive health issues such as HIV/AIDS has the potential to distort reproductive health programmes within small overworked ministries of health.

Conservative religious movements across the region lobby to block efforts to provide reproductive health services, including abortion-related care. As Hull and Widyantoro document for Indonesia in Chapter Eight, increasingly conservative Islamic politics threaten to harden Islamic interpretations of provisions in the law. They describe how abortion laws in Indonesia serve as an instrument for the harassment and manipulation of individuals. On the other hand, the Women's Health Foundation, a coalition of women's groups, obstetricians, gynaecologists and medical associations, has incorporated progressive religious groups into their discussions on reproductive health and abortion. They draw upon progress in Malaysia where interpretations of Islamic texts and a *fatwah* outlining the Islamic position on abortion demonstrate Islamic support for women's rights to contraception and abortion before ensoulment has taken place (at 120 days). They describe the frustrating attempts to reform Indonesia's restrictive abortion law and the effects of a series of ambiguous legal rulings on abortion.

Even in settings where the laws are relatively liberal such as Malaysia, fear of conservative backlash limits the dissemination of information about existing available services. In Chapter Nine, Rashidah Abdullah and Yut-lin Wong detail how abortion in Malaysia remains difficult to access. Vulnerable groups of women such as those who live in poverty, unmarried women, survivors of domestic violence or rape face discrimination and stigma when they seek abortion services. Abdullah and Wong note that modern contraceptive use remains low in Malaysia, due in part to poor promotion by the government and a lack of accessibility to quality services. Widespread misinformation about the law and beliefs that abortions are forbidden under Islam lead to women not being able to access the abortion services they are legally entitled to. Their description of institutional practices in hospitals and attitudes of medical staff highlights the truism that reform alone is not enough. The final part of this chapter outlines an agenda for action within Malaysia to ensure dissemination of information, advocacy, research and integration of abortion services within quality reproductive services.

Reform may also be conducted through indirect regulatory reforms rather than direct confrontation. The final chapter, by Nongluk Boonthai and colleagues, offers a unique first-hand account of 'activism from within': the process through which the Thai medical regulations governing abortion were reformed. Given a history of repeated political opposition to legal reform, even a small reform of the medical regulations took a number of years of painstaking lobbying, negotiations and consultation. Little has been written about the actual ways in which reform does take place, particularly what happens 'behind the scenes' in public debates, making this chapter a valuable contribution. The reforms define the interpretation of the conditions under which abortion may be legally provided, in particular clarifying the definition of 'mental health' in the law and including foetal medical conditions as criteria permitting abortion. Since this reform took place, the Thai Ministry of Public Health has begun undertaking national training of government medical staff in MVA techniques for post-abortion care to replace outdated D&C

techniques, an additional opportunity for dissemination of the new regulations to health staff. A newly formed coalition, the Women's Health and Reproductive Rights Foundation of Thailand (WHRRF), will continue to support and lobby for reform.

Conclusions

Across Asia, states actively attempt to regulate reproductive behaviours and govern populations through various interventions: campaigns to encourage smaller families, safe-sex campaigns, contraceptive distribution and laws defining the availability of abortion. These interventions stratify reproduction, defining who is empowered to reproduce and the type of families validated by the state (Ginsburg and Rapp 1995), attempting to regulate and define the reproductive intimacies of the lives and bodies of citizens. In doing so they shape the modern Asian subject, redefining the 'Asian' value of 'the family' and creating new expectations of women's productive and reproductive roles, the 'quality' of children and their care, gender relations, the experience of motherhood and fatherhood and changing filial roles. This is occurring at a time of unprecedented social change in the region, which has seen a transition from largely agricultural economies to globalised industrialisation in the last fifty years. In the past, abortion was a private act undertaken by an individual or with the assistance of family and a local skilled woman. Today, across the region, abortion has become a public concern defined and regulated by the state and is often the subject of intense national and international politics.

The chapters in this book describe some of the various consequences of these forms of governance: from family planning accessibility to laws regulating abortion, to the quality of care received in clinics. But states are not hegemonic, and this book also raises examples of forms of intervention by non-state actors: women themselves, feminist groups, religious groups, international agencies and NGO advocates attempting to modify the nature of state regulations and laws. In the midst of it all are women who find themselves facing decisions about whether to abort a pregnancy, negotiating their relationships, pragmatically weighing options for care, consulting with families, pondering moral ambiguities, seeking support and care. The degree to which women are free to make their decisions with safety depends overwhelmingly on the economic, social, cultural and legal conditions defining abortion in their country of residence.

This tension between agency and structure runs throughout the chapters of this book. Petchesky (1990: 11) suggests that the critical issue for feminists is not so much the content of women's choices, but the social and material conditions under which choices are made: 'Women make their own reproductive choices, but they do not make them just as they please; they do not make them under conditions they create but under conditions and constraints they, as mere individuals, are powerless to change'. In my previous work on abortion in northeast Thailand (Whittaker 2004), one informant in a focus group on abortion eloquently summed up the dilemma: 'Speaking very simply, poverty decides to have it [the foetus] out and start at the beginning, a new life'. In this statement, poverty is anthropomorphised as the one who makes the decision to abort. In discussions of abortions, villagers frequently spoke of how poverty 'forces' the decision; how the poor economy 'strangles' women; and how 'the situation squeezes and forces us', which also refers to massage abortion, a common technique used in that region. Such descriptions provide a stark statement of the villagers' awareness and lived experience of economic inequalities in Thai society. They identify abortion as a decision grounded in broad social and economic contexts, not just a personal decision.

To write of abortion in Asia is an inherently political act. As the authors in this volume demonstrate, to write of abortion is to expose the social and economic disparities within countries. It is to write of poverty and violence against women and the institutional violence meted out through poor services in hospitals and health centres. It exposes the operations of patriarchy within our societies. The decision to abort is enmeshed in local and global politics, which profoundly influence the experience for a woman and the safety of that act. It is a public health imperative that health services cater fully for woman's reproductive health needs, including access to abortion services when required. It is a human rights imperative that women not be denied the ability to control and decide freely about a procedure so clearly linked to their health, with legal protection, good quality care and free of discrimination and fear.

Note

1. For the most part, social science research on abortion in Asia appears in journals such as *International Studies in Family Planning*. An exception is the journal *Reproductive Health Matters,* which carries the most Asian

content on the issue from anthropological, policy and advocacy perspectives. Advocacy groups such as the Center for Reproductive Rights (2004, 2005) ARROW and Ipas (Hessini 2004) produce authoritative overviews aimed at policy-makers and donor organisations, and much Asian social science research is found in the 'grey literature' produced within countries for internal consumption and lobbying and not readily accessible to an international audience. Academic volumes on the issue have generally included few chapters on Asia, usually focused on China, Japan, or India (see Githens and McBride 1996; Mundigo and Indriso 1999). However, these volumes tend to be public health and policy oriented. Most published social science books on abortion in Asia are religious studies by Western scholars focusing on non-Western religious practices, particularly descriptions of Buddhist rituals placating vengeful foetus spirits. These include the classic book by William LaFleur, *Liquid Life: Abortion and Buddhism in Japan* (1992), and later volumes by Hardacre (1997) and Moskowitz (2001). *Buddhism and Abortion* (Keown 1998) contains chapters on a number of Buddhist countries and focuses on religious perspectives. Exceptions to this pattern include Jing Bao Nie's (2005) book on abortion in China, and my own book *Abortion, Sin and the State in Thailand* (2004), both of which offer more anthropological perspectives analysing abortion within broader social, political and ethical contexts.

References

Aahman, E. and I. Shah. 2004. *Unsafe abortion: global and regional estimates of unsafe abortions and associated mortality in 2000.* Geneva: World Health Organization.

Abeyesekera, S. 1997. 'Abortion in Sri Lanka in the Context of Women's Human Rights', *Reproductive Health Matters* 9: 87–93.

Ahmed, S., I Ariful, A. K. Parveen and Barkat-e-Khuda. 1999. 'Induced Abortion: What's Happening in Rural Bangladesh?' *Reproductive Health Matters* 7 (14): 19–29.

Ba-Thike, K. 1997. 'Abortion: A Public Health Problem in Myanmar', *Reproductive Health Matters* 9 (May): 94–100.

Belton, S. 2007. 'Borders of Fertility: Unplanned Pregnancy and Unsafe Abortion in Burmese Women Migrating to Thailand', *Health Care for Women International* 28: 419–433.

Belton, S. and A. Whittaker. 2007. 'Kathy Pan, Sticks and Pummelling: Techniques Used to Induce Abortion by Burmese Women on the Thai Border', *Social Science & Medicine* 65: 1512–1523.

Belton, S., A. Whittaker and L. Barclay. 2009. Maternal Mortality, Unplanned Pregnancy and Unsafe Abortion in Timor-Leste: A Situational Analysis. Dili: UNFPA and Alola Foundation.

Bennett, L. R. 2001. 'Single Women's Experiences of Premarital Pregnancy and Induced Abortion in Lombok, Eastern Indonesia', *Reproductive Health Matters* 9 (17): 37–43.

Berer, M. 2004. 'National Laws and Unsafe Abortion: The Parameters of Change', *Reproductive Health Matters* 12 (24) Supplement: 1–8.

Cadelina, F. V. 1999. 'Induced Abortion in a Province in the Phillipines: The Opinion, Role, and Experience of Traditional Birth Attendants and Government Midwives', in C. Indriso and M. F. Fathalla (eds), *Abortion in the Developing World.* London: World Health Organization & Zed Books, pp. 311–334.

Chu Junhong 2001. 'Prenatal sex determination and sex-selective abortion in Central China', *Population and Development Review* 27 (2): 259–281.

Center for Reproductive Rights. 2004. *Women of the World: Laws and Policies Affecting Their Reproductive Lives. South Asia.* New York: The Center for Reproductive Rights.

Center for Reproductive Rights. 2007. 'Briefing paper. Abortion Worldwide: Twelve years of reform'. http://www.reproductiverights.org/pdf/pub_bp_abortionlaws10.pdf (Last Accessed 10/9/07)

Center for Reproductive Rights, and Asian-Pacific Resource and Research Centre for Women (ARROW). 2005 *Women of the World: Laws and Policies Affecting Their Reproductive Lives. East and Southeast Asia.* New York: The Center for Reproductive Rights.

Chowdhury, S., M. Nahid and D. Moni. 2004. 'A Situation Analysis of the Menstrual Regulation Programme in Bangladesh', *Reproductive Health Matters* 12 (24) Supplement pp. 95–104.

Correa, S. 1994 *Population and Reproductive Rights: Feminist Perspectives from the South.* London: Zed Books, DAWN.

Crane, B. B. and J. Dusenberry 2004. 'Power and Politics in International Funding for Reproductive Health: The US Global Gag Rule', *Reproductive Health Matters* 12 (24): 128–137.

de Bruyn, M. 2003. *Violence, Pregnancy and Abortion. Issues of Women's Rights and Public Health.* Chapel Hill, NC: Ipas.

Delvaux, T., F. Crabbe, S. Seng and M. Laga. 2003. 'The Need for Family Planning and Safe Abortion Services among Women Sex Workers Seeking STI Care in Cambodia', *Reproductive Health Matters* 11 (21): 88–95.

Duggal, R. and V. Ramachandran. 2004. 'The Abortion Assessment Project – India: Key Findings and Recommendations', *Reproductive Health Matters* 12 (24) Supplement pp. 122–129.

Gammeltoft, T. 1999. *Women's Bodies, Women's Worries: Health and Family Planning in a Vietnamese Rural Community.* Surrey: Curzon.

Ganatra, B., M. Bygdeman, Phan Bich Thuy, Nguyen Duc Vinh and Vu Manh Loi. 2004. 'From Research to Reality: The Challenges of Introducing Medical Abortion into Service Delivery in Vietnam', *Reproductive Health Matters* 12 (24) Supplement pp. 105–113.

Ganatra, B. and H. Siddhi. 2002. 'Induced Abortions among Adolescent Women in Rural Maharashtra, India', *Reproductive Health Matters* 10 (19): 76–85.

George, S. M. 2002. 'Sex Selection/Determination in India: Contemporary Developments (Roundtable)', *Reproductive Health Matters* 10 (19): 190–191.

Ginsburg, F. D. and R. Rapp, eds. 1995. *Conceiving the New World Order: The Global Politics of Reproduction.* Berkeley, CA: University of California Press.

Githens, M. and D. McBride Stetson, eds. 1996. *Abortion Politics: Public Policy in Cross-Cultural Perspective.* London: Routledge.

Global gag rule impact project. 2003. 'Access Denied: Us Restrictions on International Family Planning'. www.globalgagrule.org

Greenhalgh, S. 2003. 'Science, Modernity, and the Making of China's One-Child Policy', *Population and Development Review* 29(2), June: 163–196.

Greenhalgh, S. and E. Winckler. 2005. *Governing China's Population: From Leninist to Neoliberal Biopolitics,* Stanford: Stanford University Press.

Gupte, M., B. Sunita and P. Hemlata. 1997. 'Abortion Needs of Women in India: A Case Study of Rural Maharashta', *Reproductive Health Matters,* 5 (9): 77–86.

Hardacre, H. 1997. *Marketing the Menacing Fetus in Japan.* Berkeley and Los Angeles: University of California Press.

Henshaw, S. K., S. Singh and T. Haas. 1999. 'The Incidence of Abortion Worldwide', *International Family Planning Perspectives* 25 Supplement: S30–S38.

Hessini, L. 2004. *Advancing reproductive health as a human right: Progress toward safe abortion care in selected Asian countries since ICPD.* Chapel Hill, NC, Ipas.

———. 2005. 'Global Progress in Abortion Advocacy and Policy: An Assessment of the Decade since ICPD', *Reproductive Health Matters* 13 (25): 88–100.

Indriso, C. and A. I. Mundigo. 1999. 'Introduction', in Indriso, C. and Mundigo, A. I. (eds) *Abortion in the Developing World.* London: World Health Organization & Zed Books, pp. 1–53.

Jing Bao Nie. 2005. *Behind the Silence: Chinese Voices on Abortion.* Lanham, MD: Rowman and Littlefield Publishers.

Keown, D. (ed.) 1992. *Buddhism and Abortion.* Honolulu: University of Hawai'i Press.

LaFleur, W. R. 1992. *Liquid Life. Abortion and Buddhism in Japan.* Princeton: Princeton University Press.

Löfstedt, P., L. Shusheng and A. Johansson. 2004. 'Abortion patterns and reported sex ratios at birth in rural Yunnan, China', *Reproductive Health Matters* 12 (24): 86–95.

Moskowitz, M. 2001. *The Haunting Foetus: Abortion, Sexuality and the Spirit World in Taiwan.* Honolulu: University of Hawai'i Press.

Nidadavolu, V. and H. Bracken. 2006. 'Abortion and Sex Determination: Conflicting Messages in Informational Materials in a District in Rural Rajasthan, India', *Reproductive Health Matters* 14 (27): 160–71.

Oaks, L. 1994. 'Fetal Spirithood and Fetal Personhood: The Cultural Construction of Abortion in Japan', *Women's Studies International Forum* 17: 511–523.

Petchesky, R. 1990. *Abortion and Woman's Choice: The State, Sexuality and Reproductive Freedom,* rev. edn., Boston: Northeastern University Press.

———. 1998. 'Introduction' in Petchesky, R. and Judd, K. (eds.) *Negotiating Reproductive Rights: Women's Perspectives across Countries and Cultures.* London: Zed Books, pp. 1–30.

Povey, G. and M. A. Mercer. 2002. East Timor in Transition: Health and Health Care-Report from East Timor. *International Journal of Health Services.* 32(3): 607–23.

Ramachandar, L. 2004. 'Decision-Making and Women's Empowerment: Abortion in a Southern Indian Community'. Ph.D. Dissertation, Key Centre for Women's Health in Society, University of Melbourne.

Ramachandar, L. and P. J. Pelto. 2002. 'The Role of Village Health Nurses in Mediating Abortions in Rural Tamil Nadu, India', *Reproductive Health Matters* 10 (19): 64–75.

———. 2004. 'Abortion Providers and Safety of Abortion: A Community-Based Study in a Rural District of Tamil Nadu, India', *Reproductive Health Matters* 12 (24) Supplement: 1–9.

———. 2005. 'Medical Abortion in Rural Tamil Nadu, South India: A Quiet Transformation', *Reproductive Health Matters* 13 (26): 54–64

Ramaseshan, G. 1997. 'Women Imprisoned for Abortion in Nepal: Report of a Forum Asia Fact-Finding Mission', *Reproductive Health Matters* 5 (10): 133–138.

Ravindran, T., K. Sundari and P. Balasubramanian. 2004. ''Yes' To Abortion But 'No' To Sexual Rights: The Paradoxical Reality of Married Women in Rural Tamil Nadu', *Reproductive Health Matters* 12 (23): 88–99.

Royal Thai Government. 2005. 'Royal Thai Medical Council regulations concerning abortion', *Royal Thai Government Gazette,* 15 December 2005:7 Book 22, Section 118g (in Thai).

Sadana, R. and R. Snow. 1999 'Balancing effectiveness, side-effects and work: women's perceptions and experiences of modern contraceptive technology in Cambodia', *Social Science and Medicine* 49: 343–358.

Shakya, G., S. Kishore, C. Bird and J. Barak. 2004. 'Abortion Law Reform in Nepal; Women's Right to Life and Health', *Reproductive Health Matters* 12 (24) Supplement: 75–84.

Singh, S. 2006. 'Hospital admissions resulting from unsafe abortion: estimates from 13 developing counties', *Lancet* 368: 18887–92.

Tamang, A. K., N. Shrestha and K. Sharma. 1999. 'Determinants of Induced Abortion and Subsequent Reproductive Behaviour Among Women in Three Urban Districts of Nepal', in Mundigo, A. and Indriso, C. (eds), *Abortion in the Developing World.* London: World Health Organization, Zed Books, pp. 167–190.

Tamang, A. and J. Tamang. 2005. 'Availability and Acceptability of Medical Abortion in Nepal: Health Care Providers' Perspectives', *Reproductive Health Matters* 13 (26): 110–119.

Tedesco, F. 1999. 'Abortion in Korea', in Keown, D. (ed.) *Buddhism and Abortion.* Honolulu: University of Hawai'i Press, pp. 121–155.

Thapa, S. 2004. 'Abortion Law in Nepal: The Road to Reform', *Reproductive Health Matters* 12 (24) Supplement: 85–94.

Thein Thein Htay, J. Sauvarin and S. Khan. 2003. 'Integration of Post-Abortion Care: The Role of Township Medical Officers and Midwives in Myanmar', *Reproductive Health Matters,* 11 (21): 27–36.

United Nations. Report of the Fourth World Conference on Women, Beijing 4–15 September, 1995. New York: United Nations, 1995.

———. Report of the International Conference on Population and Development, Cairo, 5–13 September, 1994. New York: United Nations, 1996.

United Nations 'Laos'. http://www.un.org/esa/population/publications/abortion/doc/lao.doc (2007a) (Last Accessed 10/9/07).

United Nations 'Cambodia' http://www.un.org/esa/population/publications/abortion/doc/cambod1.doc (2007b) (Last Accessed 10/9/07)

UNDP 2006 United Nations Development Programme Timore-Leste Human Development Report Path Out of Poverty Integrated Rural Development. Dili: UNDP.

Varkey, P., P. P. Balakrishna, J. H. Prasad, A. Sulochana and A. Joseph. 2000. 'The Reality of Unsafe Abortion in a Rural Community of South India', *Reproductive Health Matters* 8 (16): 83–91.

Warakamin, S., N. Boonthai and V. Tangcharoensathien. 2004. 'Induced Abortion in Thailand: Current Situation in Public Hospitals and Legal Perspectives', *Reproductive Health Matters* 12 (24) Supplement: 147–156.

Whittaker, A. 2002. 'The Struggle for Abortion Law Reform in Thailand', *Reproductive Health Matters* 10 (19): 45–53.

———. 2004. *Abortion, Sin and the State in Thailand.* New York: Routledge Curzon.

World Health Organization. 2003. *Safe Abortion: Technical and Policy Guidance for Health Systems.* Geneva: World Health Organization.

Zhou Wei-jin, Gao Er-sheng, Yang Yao-ying, Qin Fei and Tang Wei. 1999. 'Induced Abortion and the Outcome of Subsequent Pregnancy in China: Client and Provider Perspectives', in Mundigo, A. I and Indriso, C. (eds.), *Abortion in the Developing World.* London: World Health Organization & Zed Books, pp. 228–244.

Chapter Two

Contraceptive use and unsafe abortion in rural Cambodia

Elizabeth Hoban, Tung Rathavy and Phirun Lam

The Story of Oung

I was in Krasung Village this morning visiting grandmother Boeur when Sopha, a neighbour and son of the village *krue khmer* (traditional healer) also called by. Sopha asked grandmother Boeur if he could have a root of the *morom* tree that was near her house. He told us that his wife Oung was pregnant and she had miscarried the previous night. Sopha had seen the foetus and placenta expelled. He asked grandmother Boeur for three roots of the *morom* tree, as he wanted to prepare a hot herbal drink for Oung using the roots. The *morom* tree root is well known to the villagers as it is often used when postpartum women are undergoing *ang pleen* ('mother roasting', or warming) to aid in the expulsion of 'bad blood' from the uterus in the first few days after childbirth.

Grandmother Boeur told Sopha where he could dig for the roots. Sopha immediately left and went to search; within minutes, he returned with the roots in his hand. He thanked grandmother Boeur and bid us farewell. I was interested to know whom the *morom* root was for, but also why grandmother Boeur, a trained and experienced village midwife was not invited to provide post-abortion care for Oung.

Later in the afternoon I visited Sopha and Oung in their house. I remembered Oung as we had met when I was conducting household surveys, about two weeks earlier. She has four children and told me that she does not want another child. When we met, she was breast-feeding her seventeen-month-old son. Oung told us that she and another woman in the village were sharing a packet of the monthly contraceptive pills (Chinese pill). She said the market seller in Chūp Commune told her to take one pill each month and if she completed a packet of twelve tablets she would never have a pregnancy again. Oung also told me that she had not had a menstrual period for two months after having taken the Chinese pills for two months. About two weeks ago she had decided to visit the health centre and request an additional contraceptive method, the daily pill; she did not tell the health centre midwife she was taking the monthly pill. The midwife told her to wait until her menses returned before commencing the daily pill, but Oung could not wait and took the pill the same day.

A few days before Sopha's request to Grandmother Bouer, Oung had begun to think that she might be as much as three months pregnant. She had asked the 'new' midwife in the village, Grandmother Kun to massage her stomach and tell her if she was pregnant. Grandmother Kun agreed with Oung, confirming she was pregnant. Oung told grandmother Kun to continue with the deep abdominal massage and terminate the pregnancy. A few hours after the massage, Oung began to bleed from her vagina. Grandmother Kun told Oung that she was no longer pregnant. Yesterday morning, grandmother Kun had returned to Oung's house and gave her a second deep abdominal massage; the bleeding continued and in the evening Oung and Sopha had seen the foetus and placenta expelled. Oung continued to bleed overnight. This worried the couple, so early in the morning they decided to go to the private *peet* (generic term for health provider) in Chūp Commune. The private health provider gave Oung intravenous therapy, two intravenous injections, one of calcium (regarded as a hot medicine) and a second injection that Oung did not know the name of. The fee for the service was approximately US$11. Oung said that she had thought of going to the Chūp Commune Health Centre, but it was early in the morning and they could not wait for the service to open at 8 AM.

Oung told me that she felt much stronger now and that the bleeding had decreased considerably, which she put down to the injections and the root of the *morom* tree. I decided that this was a good opportunity to discuss contraceptive use with Oung. During our discussion, Oung asked me if she could keep taking the oral contraceptives. I recommended that she return to the health centre and discuss her contraceptive needs with the midwife.

(E. Hoban, fieldnotes, 21 September 2000)

Postscript: The youngest of Oung's four children is nearly eight years old and he attends the local primary school along with his two older

> brothers and sister. Oung is taking the daily pill, which she purchased from the Chūp Commune Health Centre soon after her abortion. She has taken the daily pill for more than six years and has not had a pregnancy in this time.
>
> (E. Hoban, fieldnotes, 26 February 2007)

This chapter will explore the interrelationship between contraceptive use, unwanted pregnancy and unsafe abortion in a rural Cambodian community. The story of Oung's unwanted pregnancy, her difficulty accessing modern effective contraceptives and the use of unsafe abortion techniques illustrates that, despite Cambodia's liberal abortion laws, these are common experiences for many women. The first part of this chapter explores local contraceptive knowledge and barriers to accessing modern contraceptives. The second part explores how, despite one of the most progressive abortion laws in Southeast Asia, Cambodian women continue to utilise local and often unsafe abortion services.

Setting

This chapter draws on primary data obtained by Elizabeth Hoban in 2000–2001 during a fifteen-month ethnographic study in Chūp Commune (pseudonym), Banteay Meanchey Province, northwest Cambodia. The study explored the role of *yiey maap* (grandmother midwives, hereafter referred to as grandmother) in Cambodia in the modernising health system (Hoban 2003).[1]

The women in this study are typical of the majority of rural women in Cambodia: poor, rural agricultural workers with little education. Cambodia is one of the poorest countries in Asia with a gross domestic product per capita of US$385. In 2004, 34.7 per cent of the population was living below the poverty line, estimated at US$0.59 a day for Phnom Penh residents and lower for rural residents; approximately 85 per cent of the population lives in rural areas (Cambodia, NIS 2004). A majority of households still engage in rice crop production, as many as 83 per cent in the wet season and 35 per cent in the dry season.

Forty-three per cent of women aged twenty-five years and over have no or some education (that is, have not completed first grade) compared to 20 per cent of men. Only 0.4 per cent of women and 1.8 per cent of men have post-secondary education. The adult literacy rate for those aged fifteen years and over is 60 per cent for women and 80 per cent for men. Some 3.7 million (55 per cent) of the population aged between five and twenty-four years were enrolled in the formal school system in 2004. Of the twenty to twenty-nine year old population in the labour market in 2004, 17 per cent had completed lower secondary school (Cambodia National Institute of Statistics (NIS) 2004).

Family Planning in Cambodia

Cambodia has a population of 13.5 million (Cambodia, NIS 2004) with a fertility rate of 3.4, which has decreased in both rural and urban areas in the past five years (Cambodia NIS and National Institute of Public Health (NIPH) 2006). In the Demographic and Health Survey 2005, 79 per cent of women said they either wanted to delay the birth of their next child or wanted to have no more children; these women are considered to be in need of family planning (Cambodia NIS and NIPH 2006).

Modern contraceptive use has increased over the recent past, from 19 per cent of currently married women in 2000 to 27 per cent in 2005. The increase in contraceptive use can be attributed to a desire for smaller families, increased programme activities by the Ministry of Health, National Reproductive Health Birth Spacing Programme (Cambodia's Family Planning Programme) and outreach by non-governmental organisations (NGOs) working in the reproductive health sector, community volunteer birth-spacing promoters in some rural communities, and increased knowledge and exposure to modern contraceptive methods among the wider population. Women's use of contraceptives increases steadily with increasing education. The main contraceptive methods used by Cambodian women are (in order of prevalence) the daily pill, the monthly pill (referred to as the Chinese Pill), the three monthly Depo-Provera injection, intra-uterine device (IUD), and contraceptive implants (Cambodia NIS and NIPH 2006).

Contraceptive Use and Unwanted Pregnancy

The interrelationship between contraceptive use, fertility and induced abortion is complex (Ahman and Shah 2006). Many Cambodian women express a need for contraceptive use: the 2000 Cambodian Demographic and Health Survey (Cambodia, Ministry of Planning and Ministry of Health 2001) found that while 19 per cent of currently married women were using a modern contraceptive method at the time of the study, a further one third of the women had an unmet need for contraception. This was particularly true for rural women. The Cambodia National Reproductive Health Birth Spacing Programme is one of the most developed and utilised health programmes in the country, and the increase in the contraceptive prevalence rate over the past five years can be attributed to the success of this programme. However, one of the main reasons why women's contraceptive needs are not being met is because of the spatial distance and unfavourable interpersonal relationships that exist between women in the community and the government health staff. Oung, like the majority of women in Chūp villages, has minimal contact with the government health staff, either at the health centre or during monthly outreach activities in the village; the focus of the latter is child immunisation (Hoban 2003; Vonthanak et al. 2005). There are no village-based 'information, education and communication' (IEC) programmes during outreach activities that address reproductive health: these are missed opportunities. This disjunction leads women to independently seek out contraceptive methods of unknown properties and contraindications, usually through the private sector, in order to avoid a pregnancy.

Unwanted pregnancies continue to be a problem for many women in Cambodia. They occur within a context of an increasing desire for smaller families, combined with an unmet need for family planning. Pregnancies may result from an unwanted sexual relationship; poor information, education and communication (IEC) by health providers; incorrect use of contraceptives; contraceptive failure; and confusion and miscommunication caused by local understandings of fertility and reproduction that differ from the biomedical model. Unwanted pregnancies particularly affect adolescent women, single women, and women over forty years of age. Given women's position of vulnerability, social sanctions on their sexual activity, the stigma associated with a pregnancy outside marriage, and notions of family honour and disgrace, an unsafe abortion is perceived by many women as being their only option for ending an unwanted pregnancy.

Local Understandings of Contraceptives and Fertility

In Cambodia, humoral medicine remains the basis of many indigenous beliefs about health and illness, including fertility and reproduction (Hoban 2003). Humoral medicine in Cambodia, with its intra-cultural variations and inconsistencies, is primarily based on the classification of the body and foods as hot and cold, and the elements of wind and air. The three elements that maintain internal order are phlegm, bile and blood. However, a 'simple' hot-cold dichotomy is now the dominant feature of Khmer medical beliefs, with the ranking of hot and cold by degree. The parallel classical differentiation of wet and dry has largely disappeared among the general population. Women consider the most fertile period as being just before, during and a few days after menstruation ceases (Sadana and Snow 1999; Hoban 2003): a stark contrast to Western medicine's understandings of fertility and reproduction. Women such as Oung understand that if they wait until menstruation begins before they commence a contraceptive method such as the daily pill, they can become pregnant. Women often commence a hormone-based contraceptive method when the womb is closed, such as midway through their reproductive cycle (the time Western medicine considers the most fertile period).

Cambodian women believe that hormone-based contraceptive methods such as the daily and monthly pill, and injections such as Depo-Provera can affect the humoral balance of the body: they generate internal heat in the body, which creates an unfavourable environment for fertility. Altering the body's humoral, i.e. hot-cold balance, results in the drying of the body, especially the uterus and skin, and it causes thickening of the menstrual blood (Sadana and Snow 1999; Hoban 2003). Hormone-based contraceptives in the body can make women feel weak, dizzy and internally hot. Kulig (1995:154) notes in her study with Cambodian refugee women in northern California, U.S.A., that women on hormone-based contraceptives complained of skin rashes, 'becoming skinny', losing the ability to conceive, and developing cancer.

Women believe that the daily pill generates heat in the body that then melts the man's sperm or the blood that supports the developing foetus (Sadana and Snow 1999). In comparison, three monthly hormone injections such as Depo-Provera and the monthly pill are believed to generate even more heat in the body than the daily pill, to the extent that menstruation ceases and women's skin becomes very dry, they feel lethargic and weak and develop dark pigmentation under the eyes or on the face (Khim and Saing 2003). The increase in internal heat in the body as a result of taking hormone-based contraceptive methods is thought to render the womb so weak that the foetus is unable to survive.

The IUD remains a poorly understood contraceptive method and is difficult to place in local understandings of ethno-physiology of fertility and reproduction. In Sadana and Snow's (1999) study, some women thought that the IUD 'sweeps the sperm out of the womb' while others thought that when intercourse takes place the IUD evacuates the womb. Other women felt that the IUD makes the womb open up so the sperm have to flow out of the cavity. The IUD is considered a foreign object inside the body. There is a widespread fear in Chūp villages that an IUD can leave the womb and travel throughout the body, lodging in organs such as the lungs and heart. However, women who use the IUD with success, despite not fully understanding its function, know that while it stays in the womb they will not have a pregnancy.

Traditional methods such as Khmer herbs are classified as hot and are consumed with hot water or wine, also considered hot. Khmer herbs continue to be used as a contraceptive method by some rural women, especially older multi-parity women, although their use is decreasing. Khmer herbs are believed to act in the same way as other hot contraceptive methods: by heating the body and thereby preventing fertility. Other types of Khmer herbs are routinely taken during childbirth and in the postpartum period to warm the body and maintain humoral balance as both are considered cold states (Hoban 2001; 2003). They are taken in large volumes in the postnatal period and after an abortion to facilitate the expulsion of blood from the uterus. If blood remains inside the uterus, the postpartum woman can develop life-threatening conditions such as *toah* (relapse due to loss of body heat resulting in humoral imbalance) (Hoban 2003). One Khmer herb used to expel blood from the uterus is the root of the *morom* tree. As discussed above, Sopha mixed the *morom* roots with hot water and Oung consumed several litres of the hot drink, which aided the expulsion of the foetus, placenta and blood that remained in the uterus. Khmer herbs are part of a suite of hot remedies such as *bor bor* (rice soup), along with 'mother roasting', which are routinely used by postpartum women to increase the internal heat in the body with the aim of returning the body's humours to a state of balance (Hoban 2003).

Other commonly used natural contraceptive methods are abstinence from sexual intercourse during the fertile period and withdrawal. The 2005 Demographic and Health Survey (Cambodia, NIS and NIPH 2006) found that 8 per cent of Cambodian women reported using withdrawal as a contraceptive method. Most women know that traditional methods such as Khmer herbs and withdrawal are not highly efficacious; however, they are often used in conjunction with modern methods in order to prolong the effect of modern methods, to soothe heat generated by hormone-based methods, to improve women's strength when they feel weak and to regulate women's menstrual cycle and blood flow (Sadana and Snow 1999: 348). Women in Chūp villages consider that traditional methods are more effective for inducing a miscarriage than preventing an unwanted pregnancy, a finding also noted by Sadana and Snow (1999). The majority of women have a practical rather than an ideological concern for therapies such as contraceptives and Khmer herbs, and they see nothing inconsistent in using modern and traditional medicines together.

Accessing Contraceptive Methods

Modern contraceptive methods such as the daily pill and injectable contraceptives are available in health centres throughout Cambodia at low cost (approximately US$0.30 for a three- or four-month supply), in addition to their widespread availability in pharmacies, private clinics and markets. Women in Chūp villages seeking a modern contraceptive method present to the health centre during opening hours (8 AM until 11 AM, Monday to Friday) and are seen by the primary midwife. Rarely does a secondary midwife see women regarding pregnancy and contraception in the health centre, as they are in short supply and are required to work in the District Referral Hospital. While women are aware of the health centre's opening hours, they also know that the primary midwife may not be in the health centre when they attend because she is assisting women in childbirth (either in their homes or in private clinics), providing antenatal care and immunisation services during outreach activities in the community, or busy in her private practice.

Privacy during a birth-spacing consultation in the Chūp Commune Health Centre cannot be guaranteed. The consultation takes place in a room that has two windows; neither window has curtains, and the door is never closed. Patients and their families wander in and out of the room during consultations. There can be as many as four other women sitting in the room while the birth-spacing consultation takes place. Conversely, in private clinics where government staff work privately, the patient–provider relationship is significantly different to that in the public health facilities in that women's privacy is considered.

During the birth-spacing consultation, the midwife asks the woman to provide the date for the first day of her last menstrual period. Women estimate the approximate time of their menses based on the lunar calendar, having no written record of the date or day. Women have no knowledge of the Roman calendar, and see its use as modern, scientific and outside their worldview. On the other hand, young primary midwives grow up and are trained in the use of the Roman calendar and are ignorant and dismissive of the lunar calendar used universally by Chūp villagers. Midwives often scorn women for providing lengthy details of their menstrual cycle using lunar markers. This situation invariably creates confusion when midwives try to determine the first day of a woman's last menstrual period, often resulting in the provision of inaccurate information to women as well as inaccuracies about the woman's pregnancy record.

Several problems may result from an inaccurate recording of a woman's menstrual cycle. For example, a woman may seek an abortion outside the legal limit of twelve weeks' gestation or a pregnancy may be unnoticed for some time. As noted in Oung's case, it is not routine in Chūp Health Centre for midwives to perform a physical examination to ensure that women are not pregnant prior to dispensing a contraceptive method. This is also true of private clinics, pharmacists and markets.

Many women in Chūp villages purchase contraceptive methods from the private clinic, pharmacy or market seller, which are located approximately one kilometre further along the same road as the health centre. Women pass by the health centre to go to the private providers. The majority of hormone-based contraceptive methods are available in the private sector and at comparable prices. There is a widespread belief that drugs sold in private clinics, markets and pharmacies, because they are more expensive than those sold in government health facilities, are of higher quality and more efficacious. In Oung's situation, for example, the monthly pill she purchased from a market seller came in a box with no written instructions for use in the Khmer language. The seller provided no information about the drug's properties, recommended dosage, possible side effects and contraindications. All information provided on the packet was in Chinese and the market seller does not read Chinese script. Some women purchase one or two monthly pills at a time, others share a packet of twelve tablets. Women do not routinely return to the market each month to purchase their tablet as they frequently forget, or they do not have the money for the purchase. Instead, they present days or weeks after the due date. If the market seller has sold out of the brand of Chinese pill women have been taking, women are sold another brand of the monthly pill.

Abortion in Cambodia

Cambodia has one of the highest maternal mortality ratios in Southeast Asia at approximately 437 maternal deaths to every 100,000 live births (Cambodia NIS and NIPH 2006). Maternity-related complications are one of the leading causes of death for Cambodian women aged fifteen to forty-nine years. About one in five Cambodian women who died in the seven years preceding the Demographic and Health Survey 2005 died from pregnancy related causes. It is not known how many maternal deaths result from unsafe abortions.

In 1997 the Cambodian Government revised the abortion law to allow women an elective termination of pregnancy up to twelve weeks' gestation, and for pregnancies greater than twelve weeks, an elective termination is permitted in the case of foetal abnormality or risk to the woman's life or rape (Royal Kingdom of Cambodia 1997). However, despite the legislative changes, women continue to access unsafe abortions.

The Cambodia Demographic and Health Survey 2005 (Cambodia NIS and NIPH 2006) found that 5 per cent of reproductive age women reported having one or more abortions. The majority of induced abortions occur among older women who have more than one child (Cambodia, NIS and NIPH 2006). Rural, poor and less educated women are more likely to seek an unsafe abortion and require post-abortion care than wealthier women. A 2006 survey of 110 women who attended public and private practitioners seeking an abortion found that 80 per cent of the women were married, two-thirds were employed and the majority had at least two children (Potdar et al 2008).

Forty per cent of abortions are believed to occur in the private sector. A recent study conducted in 186 public health facilities where researchers reviewed patient records over a three-week period, found that 304 women requested an abortion and 629 women attended the facilities with abortion complications over the three-week period. Of the women who requested an abortion, 54 per cent received an abortion and 46 per cent were denied services or referred to other health facilities (Fetters et al. 2006b). The mean clinical gestation of the women requesting an abortion was 9.3 weeks and more than one third of the women were in their second trimester of pregnancy. More than one third of the women were using a contraceptive method at the time of conception and one third had attempted to induce the abortion prior to presenting at the facility.

Of the women who attempted to induce an abortion, half were using a contraceptive method at the time they became pregnant. The women who tried to induce an abortion did so with the aid of a drug seller or a pharmacist (36 per cent), traditional practitioner (21 per cent), private midwife (16 per cent), public facility (10 per cent), private doctor (3 per cent) or with the aid of a relative, friend or other person (2 per cent). Twelve per cent of women tried to induce an abortion themselves at home. Women who sought initial care from drug sellers were more likely to present to public health facilities, especially low-level health centres, for abortion complications later than women who sought an abortion from a private doctor or midwife who presented to hospitals (Fetters et al. 2006b).

Oung's story highlights a range of factors that contributed to her unwanted pregnancy and massage abortion. Oung is poor, has inadequate land to grow rice and vegetables, and migrates outside the village for seasonal work. In the off-season, she runs small scale enterprises in the village; for example, she sells cooked rats for one thousand riel each (approximately US$0.25) to villagers. With four children already and still breastfeeding her seventeen-month old son, Oung and her husband decided not to have more children and opted to use the Chinese monthly pill, readily accessible in the local market. She also took the daily pill from the local health centre to ensure she did not get pregnant. However, she was already pregnant when she purchased the monthly pill and the daily pill. On both occasions Oung was not examined to determine if she was pregnant prior to being given a contraceptive method. She became alarmed when her body began to feel pregnant.

Oung's initial response was to seek out grandmother Kun, who was a 'new' grandmother midwife in Chūp villages. Grandmother Kun does not assist women in childbirth, attend village midwife training programmes, or have a relationship with the formal health system. Grandmother Kun provides massage for pregnant women to diagnose a pregnancy and when requested, she conducts deep abdominal massage to induce an abortion.

Women's abortion care seeking behaviour parallels other forms of reproductive health care, such as care during pregnancy, childbirth and the postpartum. Women are autonomous agents and are responsible for their own health and safety (Hoban 2003). They have the experiential knowledge and resources to care for themselves in their home environment, with the support of their family. Oung sought the advice of grandmother Kun, a known abortionist, and it was only when the bleeding continued that she sought the assistance of Western medicines, which are known to be quicker acting and more efficacious than traditional therapies. But once the procedure was over and the service paid for, Oung returned home and continued with her own care. Women like Oung have always relied on Khmer traditional therapies such as massage and Khmer medicines, including during the Khmer Rouge regime (1975–1979) and the years of international isolation that followed. Local knowledge systems such as humoral medicine remain intact and continue to provide women with internally consistent, effective and affordable treatments for known illnesses, such as bleeding post abortion or during childbirth. There is no reason for poor rural women such as Oung to dispense with their trusted remedies and replace them with little known, expensive and often inaccessible Western therapies.

There are twelve 'grandmother midwives' in Chūp villages and all but two women have attended the grandmother midwives' training programmes organised by the one international NGO working in the area. Grandmother midwives' contracts with women are to assist them in childbirth, not to assist women to induce an abortion. Trained grandmother midwives learn about the abortion law during the training programme. They are told by the health staff not to assist women induce an abortion because it is an illegal act to do so. No trained grandmother midwives in Chūp villages conduct abortions. As noted in Oung's story, grandmother Boeur, a trained midwife, was not called to assist Oung with her abortion and therefore had no contract with her. Instead she was asked to provide the *morom* root. Like most grandmother midwives she has extensive knowledge of Khmer herbs, especially those used in pregnancy and childbirth.

The majority of women's initial abortion care is home-based. Women seek the services of old women in the local area who specialise in massage to diagnose and terminate the pregnancy; not all villages have women with this skill. Grandmother Kun had recently arrived in Chūp villages from Tiem Kam Commune and since her arrival, many people have travelled long distances to seek her services. Sopha invited grandmother Kun to their house to determine if Oung was pregnant. Once diagnosed, Oung asked her to continue with the massage and terminate her pregnancy. The termination was successful and the foetus and placenta were expelled. Oung was responsible for her own abortion care and she therefore sought the services of a woman known to have the skill 'in the hands' to terminate the pregnancy (see similar notion in Ramachandar, this volume).

Oung's continued bleeding worried the couple, as it was more than they considered 'normal'. Early in the morning following the termination, the couple headed into Chūp Commune to seek treatment from the private health provider for the continued blood loss. Women like Oung know that private practitioners in the market centre operate twenty-four hours a day, provide most obstetric and gynaecology services that can be secured with few questions asked and at a fee that is negotiable. In doing so, they bypass the health centre. Oung said that if she had waited until 8 AM and presented to the health centre midwife she would have been 'cursed and blamed' for asking grandmother Kun to terminate her pregnancy. She also knew that if the health centre staff found out the name of the abortionist she would be located and severely reprimanded for performing an illegal act.

It is not possible to accurately estimate the time and earnings Oung lost as a result of seeking abortion care. However, based on her narrative, Oung did not engage in productive labour for approximately three days, which supports the findings of Potdar and colleagues (2008) who found that, on average, women lost 3.3 productive days work (first trimester) and 3.4 days (second trimester) as a result of seeking an abortion. Women reported losing up to 36 days of their own productive time and spending up to US$95.15 of their household income attempting to receive appropriate abortion care (Potdar et al. 2008). This is a significant amount of money when one considers that more than one third of the Cambodian population lives on or below the poverty line (Cambodia NIS 2004). Women who visited government hospitals, health centres or private midwives lost the least amount of productive work time, compared to women who went to private and NGO clinics, 3.6 and 6.9 days, respectively. The number of lost days varied by the type of uterine evacuation procedure. Abortion clients reported losing 2.4 and 2.3 days for dilatation and curettage and medication abortions respectively. In comparison, women who received procedures using vacuum aspiration methods lost 3.6 days, and with the Kovac's procedure to induce contractions it was 23.3 days of lost time in productive work.[2]

Oung's post-abortion care from the private health provider consisted of intravenous therapy, two injections, one of calcium and the other was unknown to Oung, at a cost of 39,000 Riel (approximately US$10). She did not receive a uterine evacuation procedure. Following this, Oung and Sopha sought Khmer herbs from grandmother Boeur. Sopha prepared the *morom* root by mixing it with hot water. Oung wrapped her body in layers of warm clothing and a headscarf and consumed litres of the Khmer herbal drink along with several bowls of hot rice soup. The ultimate goal of this home-based treatment was to return the hot-cold balance of the body, which would facilitate the expulsion of the blood that remained inside the uterus. Women using traditional methods drink litres of Khmer herbs for weeks after an abortion.

Conclusions

The events that had transpired over the three-day period had a profound impact on Oung and Sopha, and they were left resolute that they would not experience another unwanted pregnancy and abortion again. Oung presented to the health centre and met with the midwife soon after the abortion. She did not tell the midwife about her pregnancy and abortion, as she feared she would be verbally abused by the midwife and that grandmother Kun would be implicated in the abortion. Oung requested and was given the daily pill and information about the use of this contraceptive method. As noted from the postscript, Oung has continued to use the daily pill for more than six years without a pregnancy.

Oung's story highlights the interrelationships between barriers to women's access to modern contraceptives, the experience of unwanted pregnancies and the use of unsafe abortion techniques. Oung attempted to access modern contraceptives, but poor quality of care at the public health service contributed to her pregnancy being missed by the service provider. Without widespread understanding of Cambodia's abortion legislation, and within a Theravadan Buddhist cultural context where abortion is still considered sinful and secretive, women rarely discuss the subject of abortion with health providers or other women; many still believe that abortion is illegal in Cambodia (Hoban 2003). Moreover, the government is slow to provide guidance for public-sector provision of abortion services with guidelines yet to be forthcoming. Fetters and colleagues' study (2006a) with primary maternity care providers in government health facilities found that only one fifth of the respondents knew that the Cambodian abortion law allows for first trimester abortions on request. Nearly half the participants thought that abortion was legal only in the case of danger to a mother's life. Of some concern, is that the majority of health care providers felt that the abortion rate in Cambodia has increased and that it is due to heightened promiscuity and women's carelessness with contraceptive use. Therefore, they believed that improving access to abortion services would only increase sexual promiscuity. The respondents felt that abortion services should only be available to women that are trying to use a contraceptive method. Half the government health staff interviewed felt that termination on social and economic grounds was not justifiable.

The legalisation of abortion in Cambodia has not resulted in increased access to safer abortion and post-abortion care. While the legislation is in place, abortion services have been slow to eventuate in the public sector. Yet they are widely available and unregulated in the private sector. Forty-seven per cent of hospitals, 10 per cent of high-level health centres, and 5 per cent of low-level health centres provide elective abortion services with wide variation in the cost of the services (Rathavy et al. 2006). The main reasons for not providing elective abortion services in government health facilities have been determined to be the lack of training of health staff and inadequate supplies. However, staffs' negative attitude towards women seeking an elective abortion is also widespread, especially towards adolescents who often find that abortion care is unavailable to them (Rathavy et al 2006:20). Generally, government health staff are not aware that abortion is legal and under what circumstances it is legal. Those that do are unclear about the detail and are often reluctant to perform elective abortions for fear of reprisal by authorities.

Government health staff that do provide abortion services are frequently not trained in safe abortion or post-abortion care, have had limited experience of the procedure and do so covertly. Therefore, it is not surprising that women such as Oung consider abortion to be illegal and inaccessible and may spend days seeking out an abortion provider. This situation leads to many delays in accessing abortion care, increased costs and loss of productive days. Such delays often result in the abortion being conducted by an untrained and unskilled abortion provider, which influences rates of maternal morbidity and mortality. In Oung's case, she was fortunate not to experience serious complications from her massage abortion and sought and received contraceptive advice. Until access to contraceptives and safe abortion is improved in Cambodia and there is recognition of the context of pluralistic care-seeking and local understandings of the actions of contraceptives and abortion, women such as Oung will continue to risk their health and lives with unsafe abortions.

Notes

1. Data was obtained from four villages with a total population of 1,575 people, in particular from key informant interviews with government and private-sector health providers, grandmother midwives, case studies of nine grandmother midwives, participant observations and in-depth interviews with thirty women on multiple occasions during their pregnancy, birth and postpartum period.
2. A Kovac's procedure is a technique involving the instillation of extra-amniotic saline to induce contractions and subsequent abortion in a pregnancy between sixteen and twenty weeks LMP (see list of terms).

References

Ahman, E. and I. Shah. 2006. 'Contraceptive use, fertility and unsafe abortion in developing countries', *The European Journal of Contraception and Reproductive Health Care* 11 (2): 126–131.

Cambodia, National Institute of Statistics. 2004. *Cambodia Socio-Economic Survey.* Phnom Penh: Ministry of Planning.

Cambodia, National Institute of Statistics & National Institute of Public Health. 2006. *Cambodia Demographic and Health Survey 2005.* Phnom Penh: Ministry of Health.

Cambodia, Ministry of Planning and Ministry of Health. 2001. *Cambodia Demographic and Health Survey 2000.* Phnom Penh: Ministry of Planning, National Institute of Statistics & Ministry of Health, Directorate General for Health.

Fetters. T., T. Rathavy, S. Vonthanak, C. Picardo, S. Vannat and L. Phirun. 2006a. *Don't ask, don't tell: Breaking the silence surrounding abortion among maternity care providers in Cambodia.* Research Brief. Phnom Penh: Ministry of Health, National Reproductive Health Programme & Ipas.

Fetters, T., S. Vonthanak, T. Rathavy and C. Picardo. 2006b. *A national assessment of the magnitude and consequences of abortion and abortion complications in Cambodia.* Research Brief. Phnom Penh: Ministry of Health, National Reproductive Health Programme & Ipas.

Hoban, E. 2003. 'We're safe and happy already. Traditional birth attendants and safe motherhood in a rural Cambodian commune'. Ph.D. dissertation. Melbourne: Key Centre for Women's Health in Society, Department of Public Health, Faculty of Medicine, Dentistry and Health Sciences, The University of Melbourne.

Khim, S. and H. Saing. 2003. *Perceptions and Experiences of Users and Suppliers of the Monthly (Chinese) Pill in Phnom Penh.* Working Paper No.6. Phnom Penh: Centre for Population Studies, Royal University of Phnom Penh and United Nations Family Planning Programme.

Kulig, J. C. 1995. 'Cambodian refugees' family planning knowledge and use', *Journal of Advanced Nursing* 22: 155–157.

Potdar, R., T. Fetters and L. Phirun. 2008. 'Initial Loss of Productive Days and Income Among Women Seeking Abortion in Cambodia', *Journal of Midwifery and Women's Health* 53 (6): 123–129.

Rathavy, T., T. Fetters, J. Sherman and S. Vonthanak. 2006. *Ready or not? A national needs assessment of abortion services in Cambodia.* Ministry of Health, National Reproductive Health Programme and Ipas. Phnom Penh: Ministry of Health and IPAS.

Royal Kingdom of Cambodia. 12 November 1997. Unpublished translation of the *Kram* on Abortion: Phnom Penh.

Sadana, R. and R. Snow. 1999. 'Balancing effectiveness, side-effects and work: women's perceptions and experiences of modern contraceptive technology in Cambodia,' *Social Science and Medicine* 49: 343–358.

Vonthanak, S., S. Leang, R. Leang, A. Erpelding and E. Hoban. 2005. *Report on the Evaluation of the Outreach Activities Applied Research Kampot Province. Report to the German Technical Cooperation Support to the Health Sector Reform Programme and Cambodia, Ministry of Health.* Phnom Penh: Ministry of Health & National Institute of Public Health.

Chapter Three

Between Remembering and Forgetting

Maintaining Moral Motherhood after Late-Term Abortion

Tine M. Gammeltoft

Between 2003 and 2006 I got to know a number of women living in Vietnam's capital, Hanoi, who opted to terminate a wanted pregnancy because the foetus had been diagnosed through an ultrasonography as 'abnormal'. In this chapter I examine how women and their relatives sought to come to terms with this unsettling experience in ways that enabled them to maintain personal and familial moral virtue while also protecting the woman's future reproductive capacities.

In present-day Vietnam, obstetrical ultrasound scanning and other technologies for prenatal diagnosis are proliferating, becoming increasingly routinised parts of pregnancy care (Gammeltoft 2007a). As a consequence of this mass screening, growing numbers of pregnant women are informed that the child they expect fails to live up to biomedical definitions of 'normality'. This development has given decisions surrounding abortion a new twist, as women and their relatives must decide whether to continue or to terminate 'affected' pregnancies, even at advanced stages of gestation.[1] Post-diagnostic abortions differ from most other pregnancy terminations in at least two key respects: they are obtained by women who had planned and wanted the child they expected, and they are performed on the background of complex deliberations regarding what 'normality' means and where to set the limits for entry into the human community (cf. Gammeltoft 2007b; Gammeltoft et al. 2008; Rapp 1999).[2]

Separation is a universal existential given (Stafford 2003). In all societies, people have developed a range of communal and ritual ways of responding to death and other forms of loss (eg. Bloch and Parry 1982; Feuchtwang 2003; Hertz 1907; Huntington and Metcalf 1979). But in losing a child that they had not yet had, the women I got to know in Vietnam found themselves in a culturally unprecedented predicament. The loss they experienced was ridden with ambiguities; their 'child' was not yet fully a child; its 'birth' was also a death; and the defectiveness of its body brought into question not only the child's own personhood but also the moral habitus of its kin group (cf. Gammeltoft 2007b). The loss they suffered was rendered particularly painful by having been 'chosen' by the women and their relatives themselves. In a country where mothering is culturally and politically celebrated and defined through virtues such as selflessness and loving care for others (Pashigian 2002; Pettus 2003; Phinney 2005), giving up motherhood at a late stage of pregnancy is a morally challenging act. In this situation, women and their relatives pondered questions such as: Should parents commemorate the soul of a child that had not yet been born, or should they ignore it and relegate it to oblivion? Should an anomalous foetus be treated as a thing or as a human being, as an unwelcome intruder or as a beloved family member? Young women and their senior relatives often differed radically in their immediate responses to such questions: the women who underwent abortions often described themselves as eager to 'remember' the child they had lost through commemorative rituals, whereas their senior relatives insisted that the child must be forgotten.

In this chapter I argue that the family tensions that arose indexed not only disagreements regarding the ontological status of the deceased foetus – was it a child, a potential child, a spirit, a monster? – but also and primarily uncertainties regarding how to maintain moral virtue when confronting a highly unsettling loss of a potential family member. At stake were different moral agendas: for the women, it was important to establish moral virtue by acting as loving mothers to the child they had lost; yet for their elders, protection of the younger woman's reproductive capacities was paramount. In practice, these two sets of agendas intersected and collided when families had to decide how to handle the foetal body after the abortion.

To begin with, I shall introduce 23-year-old Vân.[3] Vân was one of the pregnant women involved in the research on the use of obstetrical ultrasonography for prenatal screening that my Vietnamese colleagues and I conducted in Hanoi and surrounding provinces.[4] She lived with her husband Vinh in his parents' house in an inner-city district where my colleague Hằng and I visited them on 27 April 2004. Three weeks earlier, Vân had undergone an abortion in her twenty-first week of pregnancy after an ultrasound scanning had found abnormal amounts of fluid in the body of the foetus.

Living With Loss: The Moral Ambiguities of Abortion for Foetal Anomaly

When Hằng and I arrived, a middle-aged woman was waiting for us. This was Vân's mother-in-law, Bà Xìn. She led us through the grocery store she ran at the ground floor of their house, selling biscuits, cookies, candy and soft drinks, and up the narrow stairs to the top floor where Vân and Vinh lived. On the way, she explained that her daughter-in-law still spent most of her time in bed, recovering from the abortion.

Vân was pale and spoke in a quiet voice. She began her story by telling us – in a manner that was unusually open, given the sensitivity of the topic – that when she became pregnant she was still unmarried. This was her second pregnancy. The first time she got pregnant, two years earlier, she had an induced abortion at about seven weeks' gestation. She emphasised that she had only made this decision because she was strongly encouraged by her friends and by Vinh to terminate the pregnancy: since she was still a student, they had told her, she could not yet have a child. But for Vân herself this had been an agonising choice:

> After the abortion I could not stop thinking about the fact that I had given up a foetus (*một cái thai*), I felt it was wrong (*tội lỗi*). I kept thinking of it and felt very depressed. I felt I was a bad person, I was so sad and I did not want to live anymore … I felt I had thrown away a human being. I felt that life had no meaning anymore. It was as if my entire life was a failure.

When Vân became pregnant again, she was happy to know that her first abortion had not rendered her infertile, and this time she wanted to carry the pregnancy to term. She and Vinh therefore informed their parents that they intended to get married and have the child. Both sets of parents fiercely opposed the idea of marriage, arguing that a premarital pregnancy would ruin the reputations of their families. Their fathers tried to force her to go into hospital to terminate the pregnancy, but she fled, and eventually their parents accepted the marriage and their plans to keep the pregnancy.

Vân was three months pregnant when she and Vinh got married. Two months later, an ultrasound scan revealed that the foetus was 'not normal'. They discussed the problem with their families, and everyone immediately agreed that the best solution was a termination of the pregnancy. The abortion was performed by inducing labour, and the foetus was dead at delivery. Vân described this as a profound loss. She described the emotional emptiness she felt and the pain of seeing other mothers in the maternity ward care for their newborns, while she herself had no child to take care of: 'At the hospital, there were many women in my room and many of them had their babies there too. Seeing them made me so sad. When they went home they felt happy and carefree, and they had a child to bring home. But I had no child'. In this situation of emotional distress, Vân still tried to act in a 'motherly' fashion towards the child she had lost – the foetus was dead, she said, but what she *could* do was to at least ensure that it was properly buried. Her mother and other members of her natal family supported her in this: 'I thought it was better to take it home and bury it. I felt it would be a pity for my child if it were not buried. My [natal] family also told me to bring it home. In my family we take spiritual matters quite seriously and I often go to the pagoda to pray'. Yet her mother-in-law intervened, telling Vân to leave the foetal body at the hospital. This dilemma regarding how to handle the deceased foetal body became a source of family controversy to a much larger extent than the decision to terminate the pregnancy had been. Whereas everyone in both kin groups had immediately agreed that an abortion was necessary, the question of how to handle the foetal remains became a matter of heated family debate and disagreement.

Across the world, the ending of a human life is interpreted and handled through bereavement rituals that guide people through the first difficult period after a death has occurred. Yet some deaths are harder than others for people to handle. Untimely deaths tend to challenge conventional commemorative orders: 'The body that experiences a bad death – the untimely death of a child, for instance ... signifies not only an absence of regenerative potential but also a threat to social continuity' (Kwon 2006: 14). In Vietnam, a bad death is defined by factors such as dying young, childless, in a violent manner or in a way that leaves the body incomplete (Malarney 2003: 59). The deaths experienced by women in Vân's situation were bad deaths in more than one sense: they were untimely, taking place very early in the life of a potential child, and they were the results of violent and deliberate human interventions in reproductive processes. One young man, whose wife had an abortion at twenty-two weeks' gestation, described the moral problems at issue in these terms: 'I feel pity for the little one. It is a living being, it is immoral to abort it. This is a question of family morality. To terminate this pregnancy is equal to killing a person … To have to make this decision oneself makes me feel very uncomfortable morally. I feel very troubled'.

The tension between the decision that the women and their families had made and culturally powerful ideals of the selfless, self-sacrificing, caring mother was, however, something that came up mainly in indirect ways in our meetings with the women; it was, it seemed, an issue that was too painful to be broached directly in conversation. When I asked one woman, Châu, what she had been thinking of on the day preceding her abortion, she replied, 'It is very difficult to say aloud. Let me write it down for you'. In my notebook she wrote: *'cảm thấy có tội với con, làm thế là mình tước đi quyền được sống, được làm người của nó'* (I feel I have done wrong towards my child. Doing this means that I take away its right to live, to become a person). The abortion decision, it seemed, was a failure of motherhood so deep that it could hardly be articulated. What could be articulated, in contrast, were the good reasons that women and their relatives had to opt for a pregnancy termination. Usually, as in Vân's case, the entire family concurred that, for the child's own sake, the pregnancy could not be maintained. In family deliberations, the abortion was framed as an act that spared the child from the suffering it would have had to endure if it were born disabled (Gammeltoft et al. 2008). Still, the abrupt termination of their pregnancy left the women in a morally challenging situation where they sought to make sense of their choice in ways that allowed them to maintain moral virtue as potential mothers. In this situation, many stated that they wanted to 'remember' the child they had lost through commemorative rituals of incense burning and prayers.[5]

However, as Vân's case illustrates, when mothers-to-be sought to demonstrate maternal affection through ritual commemoration, senior relatives often intervened and stopped them from doing so. To understand what turned commemorative rituals into a terrain of conflict and contestation within families, I shall now look more closely at death rituals in Vietnam.

'To Bury the Dead Means to Create a New House for Them': Death Rituals in Vietnam

In a classic essay, Robert Hertz (1907) drew on ethnographic data from Southeast Asia to explore how social collectivities grapple with the loss of one of their members. Writing in the universalising vein characteristic of the social sciences of his time, he emphasised that death is much more than a physical event:

> But where a human being is concerned the physiological phenomena are not the whole of death. To the organic event is added a complex mass of beliefs, emotions and activities which give it its distinctive character. We see life vanish but we express this fact by the use of a special language: it is the soul, we say, which departs for another world where it will join its forefathers. The body of the deceased is not regarded like the carcass of some animal: specific care must be given to it and a correct burial; not merely for reasons of hygiene but out of moral obligation (1907: 27).

As Hertz observed, death is often a lengthy state of passage from the world of the living to the world of ancestors, and human responses to the shock of death often centre on the materiality of the body: 'The material on which the collective activity will act after the death, and which will be the object of the rites, is naturally the very body of the deceased ... It is the action of society on the body that gives full reality to the imagined drama of the soul' (1907: 83). In Vietnam too, funeral rites centre on the dead person's body. In order to ensure the passage of the soul of the deceased into the 'other world', careful ritual preparation of the body is essential (cf. Kwon 2006; Malarney 2002, 2003). Until a series of elaborate rites have been performed, the soul exists in a liminal space where it risks turning into a restless ghost rather than a family ancestor. Ideally, three years after the death a secondary burial ceremony (*bốc mộ*) should be held where the bones of the deceased are cleaned and reburied and relatives meet for a commemorative feast. Completing this secondary burial enables the soul of the deceased to end its passage into the 'other world' and become a family ancestor.[6] As Kwon writes, 'this' and 'the other' world constitute two different spheres of existence, yet they are intimately intertwined in daily lives: 'Vietnamese popular culture emphasises the supreme importance of remembering the dead, but its emphasis is on the dead person's *living* presence rather than the memory of this person' (2006: 63). Although it was questioned during the socialist revolution where state efforts were made to replace 'superstition' by 'science' (Gammeltoft 2002; Malarney 2002), the notion of souls (*linh hồn*) remains centrally placed in Vietnamese popular culture, and deceased family members continue to play important roles in the social lives of the living. When we talked about differences between Vietnamese people and foreigners, Vân linked Vietnamese cultural identity directly to the belief in souls:

> In Vietnam, people often believe in souls and many other thoughts spring from this, compelling us to take moral matters seriously. In Buddhism there is a strong moral tradition, stating for instance that abortion is wrong. But foreigners rarely think about the soul. If they have an abortion they will simply have another child. They look at it in a more scientific way.

The notion of souls indexes a particular view of human life and personhood: when the people we met reflected on human existence, they often defined life in terms that extended it beyond the material, physical world into the 'other world' of ghosts and spirits. In the homes we visited, the presence of the dead was striking. The ancestral altar was usually placed at the centre of the house, taking up a prominent position and decorated with incense sticks in pots, flowers and fruits – the amounts and kinds varying depending on the calendar day and on the economic means and ritual devotion of the family (Jellema 2007). On the altar or the wall above it were often displayed photographs or portraits of deceased elders who, during important life events such as weddings, births or deaths, were drawn into the family circle through prayers and incense burning. Vân described to us how the dead are included in the intimate domestic worlds of the living:

> To bury the dead means to create a new house for them. It means that they will be worshipped (*thờ cúng*) within the family, that the living will think of them and sometimes burn incense for them. When one burns incense there is also always fruit and rice. So it means that one does not need to feel pity for the deceased, as they are still remembered and not abandoned down in the other world (*cõi âm*).

In many houses, a smaller altar was established in addition to the central ancestral altar, in commemoration of someone who died before reaching parenthood and/or old age, such as a sister or brother

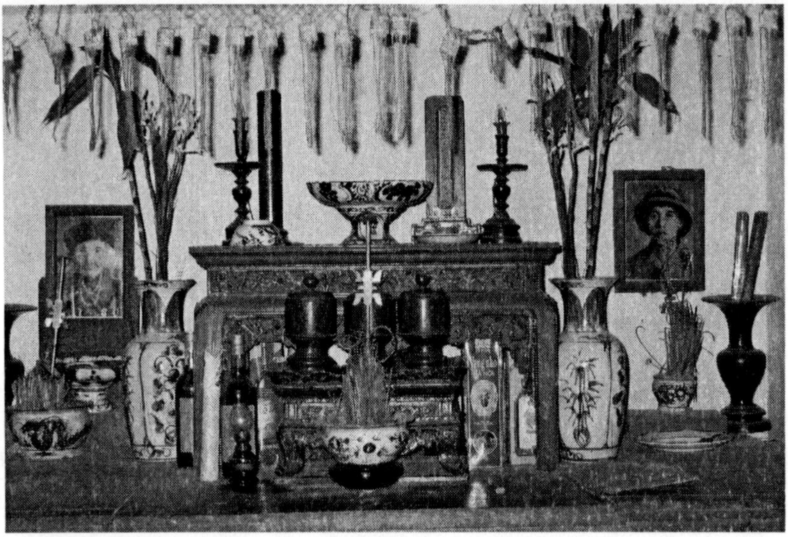

ILLUSTRATION 3.1 An ancestral altar, Bắc Ninh province (Photograph: T Gammeltoft).

who perished during the 'American' War. But not all of a family's dead were visibly and materially commemorated (cf. Kwon 2006). During our visits to families in and around Hanoi we heard many stories of deceased family members in whose memory no rites were performed and for whom no domestic memorials were erected: those who died before reaching adulthood. Child deaths, being genealogically disorderly, often seemed to be associated with considerable ambiguity.[7] People told us that death rituals held for children, while varying according to local tradition, are generally much simpler than those for adults: children are most often buried immediately after death, and in the recent past they were usually simply rolled in a mat rather than placed in a coffin. Annual commemoration on the day of their death is conducted through minimal ritual observance, if at all, and no secondary burials are held, as the bones of small children are said to be so soft that they will have disintegrated before three years have passed. As one elderly woman explained when we talked about the deaths of children,

> A child has to be able to walk and to have a name before we worship it, offering it rice and eggs and inviting it home to eat. Only when a child can say 'grandma', 'grandpa' would we worship it. Worshipping means to offer food, but a young child cannot eat at all. If it cannot yet talk it goes to another house, or to a pagoda. Those who have no one worshipping them go to pagodas.

In the stories we heard about social responses to child death, dead infant children were defined as marginal to the kin group and the domestic sphere; rather than being ritually incorporated among ancestors worthy of commemoration, efforts seemed to be made to erase them from collective social memory. The social existence of young children, in other words, was defined as tentative and evanescent, turning the child's being into a more 'fluid' form of life. In his historical study of abortion and Buddhism in Japan, William LaFleur (1992) describes how Buddhist beliefs regarding the beginning and ending of life are structured by the notion of 'return': at death, foetuses, infants and young children are held to return to 'the other world' that they came from. From there, they may later return to the present world; a thought that provides consolation for those who experience child loss. The simplicity of death rituals for children, LaFleur maintains, should be seen in this context: by keeping rituals simple, children's relatives seek to facilitate their rebirth into this world, whereas elaborate rituals would 'urge the infant too far out of reach and out of mind' (1992: 27; see also Oaks 1994). Similarly, on the topic of infant deaths, Hertz writes: 'Indeed, since the children have not yet entered the visible society, there is no reason to exclude them from it slowly and painfully. As they have not really been separated from the world of spirits, they return there directly, without any sacred energies needing to be called upon, and without a period of painful transition appearing necessary' (1907: 84).

But if the social lives of young children are tentative and fragile, and their deaths only temporary, then what kind of social status is ascribed to children-to-be who are still in the womb? A newly deceased foetus is doubly liminal: positioned in between life and death, the human and the not-yet-human (cf. Douglas 1966). A malformation triples this liminality, placing the anomalous foetus uneasily between the human and the monstrous (cf. Layne 2003). For the people we met, this liminal and ambiguous status of the foetus raised vexed questions concerning how to respond ritually to its death.

The Power of Spirits: Countering Risks of Recurrence

'Will you take the little one home afterwards', I asked Châu on a morning in March 2004. We were at the obstetrics hospital, and Châu, who was seventeen weeks pregnant, was scheduled to undergo an abortion later in the day. I was sitting at her bedside while

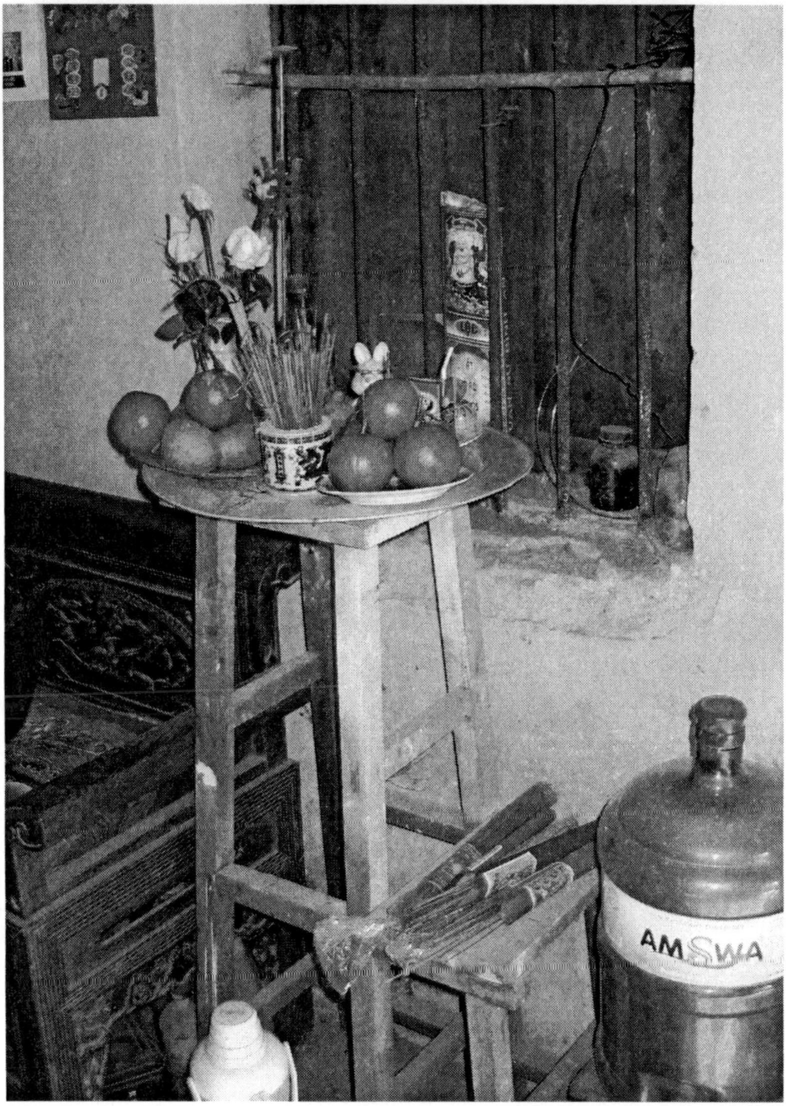

ILLUSTRATION 3.2 An altar for a deceased girl, Hanoi (Photograph: T Gammeltoft).

she was eating a plate of rice and meat that her husband had brought for her, and we were talking about what was going to happen now. At my question, Châu looked bewildered, then reached resolutely into her pink plastic handbag, which she had placed on her bedside table, grabbed her mobile phone and dialled a number. After a few minutes she ended the call and told me that she had talked to her father in Hà Tĩnh province, 300 kilometres south of Hanoi. He had told her not to worry: he and her elder brother would make the long trip to the obstetrics hospital in Hanoi to collect the body of the foetus and take it home to bury at the family's gravesite.

A range of ideas and practices suggests that early human life is often afforded considerable social significance in Vietnam. The term for 'being pregnant' is *có thai*, to 'have a foetus'. At birth, infants are usually regarded as being one year old, as the nine months of gestation are counted as the first year of life. When we asked them at what stage of gestation the foetus is considered to have a soul, people would often point to the moment when it achieves a 'human form' (*hình người*), approximately four months into a pregnancy. Most people also maintained that at death, foetal souls do not travel to 'the other world' and settle there among other deceased family members; yet there were varying opinions about where they go instead.[8] Some said that the soul would pass over to 'some other world', a kind of limbo, where it would live together with other malformed foetuses like itself; some imagined that it would hang around at a pagoda or another place of worship; and some claimed that it would reincarnate (*đầu thai*) and be born again, either to the same or to another woman, this time possibly making a more auspicious entry into the world in an 'intact' (*lành lặn*) body.[9] But a shared assertion in the majority of the familial deliberations that we witnessed was that a second trimester foetus, although unborn and malformed, must still be regarded as a human being with a life of its own (*một kiệp người*).[10] The term that people used, *kiệp*, belongs to Buddhist terminology, where it refers to each life in a series of reincarnations. Most abortion-seeking women insisted that because the foetus was a human being, they had a moral obligation to ensure that 'decent' (*đàng hoàng*) burial rites were held. Often there was also a more pragmatic edge to these moral deliberations: if the foetal body was not decently buried, women explained, the foetal soul might keep haunting them, feeling resentment (*oán*) against their families for not allowing it to live. As a restless and angry spirit, the foetal soul might cause problems such as maternal mental imbalances or illnesses in the family's children. A proper funeral, women reasoned, was therefore an important way of appeasing the foetal spirit and curbing the resentment it might feel (see also Gammeltoft 2003; LaFleur 1992; Moskowitch 2001; Hardacre 1997).

Yet despite the consensus on the importance of a decent burial, only half of the families eventually brought the foetus home with them, while the other half left it at the hospital.[11] Often, doubts lingered among women and their relatives regarding whether the hospital would *really* conduct these rites. As Vân said, 'My mother described how they would bury it at the hospital. They would collect all the children without families in one place and burn them to ashes. I thought it sounded dreadful, so at first I wanted to take it home'. In situations like this, health staff would reassure their patients that burial rites were certainly conducted with care by hospital staff. As Dr. Lan, a senior obstetrician, explained:

> If the foetus is so big that it has a human form, we do treat it very carefully. We put it into a pretty coffin and we also offer prayers, everything. We do it very decently. It is brought to the graveyard by a car from the funeral house, which comes here every day. The only difference is that the graves are not numbered as for adults, so that later one does not know exactly where it was buried.

But if a decent burial is of such importance, what then compelled half of the families to place the responsibility for this burial in the hands of strangers, rather than at the heart of their family, as normally occurs when someone dies?

All the women we met expressed acute anxiety at the thought that their next pregnancy might go awry too. This anxiety was shared by their relatives, and particularly by their husbands' parents who depended on the childbearing capacities of their daughter-in-law for continuation of the patrilineage (cf. Oosterhoff et al. 2008).[12] In this context, where both the woman's personal fulfilment and the continuation of the lineage were at stake, women and their families drew direct connections between death rituals and the risk of recurrence. Ancestor worship in Vietnam is highly localised, and death rituals, when properly conducted, tie the deceased to the dwellings of the living. Caring for the souls of the dead therefore has social consequences, as souls become attached to the place where they are worshipped. When elderly family members die, this attachment is desired by the family, as it supports bonds of love, intimacy and mutual assistance between the living and the dead. But when a malformed foetus died, detachment rather than attachment became socially and ritually paramount: it was fear of attaching the foetal soul to their family that compelled senior relatives to discourage abortion-seeking women from commemorating the deceased foetus. In this way, they sought to exorcise the foetal spirit from the body of the family, arguing that if the mother revealed her love for the child-to-be by ritually addressing it, it would keep 'hanging around' and haunting them.[13] As Dr. Lan explained:

> If you take the foetus home you must establish an altar and commemorate the day of death, and then it will hang around (*luẩn quẩn*). Therefore people ask the hospital to take care of this. When it's over, it's over (*xong là xong thôi*). You don't need to remember the day or burn incense, it is like an early miscarriage. In this way, our traditions support mothers.

The abortion-seeking women were therefore caught in a morally challenging situation where they wanted to enact maternal care through incense burning and prayers – while also being compelled by their elders to forget and let go. These contradictory forces lingered in Vân's description of her own practices of commemoration:

> I think I can remember without burning incense, I can remember in my heart. I always think about it and remember it, so I do not need to feel so much pity for it. Burning incense makes you feel sadder because you burn incense for the dead, but I don't burn incense, I just think about a little one that was not yet born. Later I will have another child and perhaps this child will jump into the body of the next child.

None of the abortion-seeking women, and very few of their husbands, took part in the burial of the deceased foetus, as their relatives told them that this would only deepen their attachment to the foetus, making it harder for them to overcome their loss. Most of the women also followed their elders' advice and refrained from including the foetus within the domestic domain by commemorating it at the ancestral altar through incense burning, prayers or offerings. But there were exceptions. Hương's abortion was completed on the first day of the lunar month and she therefore intended to include the foetus among all those she had in mind when burning incense on this day. Hạnh regularly burnt incense in commemoration of the foetus at a Buddhist pagoda, an institution that seems to embrace socially marginal beings and disruptive life events more easily than many other institutions in Vietnamese society (Kwon 2006: 71). Thủy told us that she intended to burn incense for this foetus when she commemorated her ancestors at their death anniversaries, while Nga planned to buy children's clothes made from paper to burn on the 15th day of the seventh lunar month, the day of 'wandering souls' (*linh hồn lang thang*), when people commemorate 'lost' souls. Nga explained how she had come to place the foetus in the category of 'wandering souls' rather than in that of 'family members': 'When I came home from the hospital, I intended to burn incense and to buy some clothes to burn. But my parents-in-law did not like the idea, they were afraid that [if I did so] it would hang on forever, so eventually I didn't'.

Nearly all of the women and their relatives were concerned about the implications of the abortion for the mother's future health and fertility, but not all were equally concerned about the disruptive powers of the foetal spirit, and some saw beliefs in lingering foetal souls and repeated rebirths as 'merely superstition'. They too feared a foetal 'return', but by this, they maintained, they referred to the foetus becoming a continuous psychological presence in its parents' lives, a mental phantom that would haunt them and disturb their peace of mind. For women in particular, we were told, mental obsession with a lost child can have grave consequences, as sadness and depression during pregnancy is widely believed to cause reproductive harm. So when Bà Xìn, like other senior relatives, advised her daughter-in-law to leave the foetus at the hospital, she did this with Vân's future childbearing in mind. Eventually this line of reasoning convinced both Vân and her mother to leave the foetal body at the hospital:

> My mother-in-law was concerned that if we worshipped it at home, we would often think about it and this would affect us psychologically. Therefore, she found it better to leave it at the hospital. At first my mother did not agree. She said that if my parents-in-law rejected the little one, then she would take it home and bury it. But when I explained to her that my mother-in-law was concerned about our future mental well-being, she too accepted the decision to leave it at the hospital … It would have been good if I could bury my child, but I am a very sensitive person and I am afraid that worshipping it would make me think too much about it.

In sum, when senior relatives opted to leave the foetal body at the hospital, they did so out of fear that a burial at the family gravesite would attach the foetus to its family and particularly to its mother, causing future reproductive distress. Through 'decent' burial rites – conducted either by relatives or by hospital staff – women therefore sought to attain the difficult balance between demonstrating maternal care for the child they had lost and bringing the family's involvement with this potentially dangerous spiritual being to an end.

Between Remembering and Forgetting: A Vietnamese *ars memoria*

Feeling insecure and anxious about their reproductive futures, young women such as Vân were often willing to listen to their elders' advice; and in many cases, their own mothers and mothers-in-law had only too much personal experience with reproductive loss upon which to draw when counselling a younger woman. Vân's mother-in-law, for instance, had lost her first two children shortly after birth. They were born one year apart, both at seven months' gestation, and died at the hospital. During our talk with Vân, Bà Xìn joined our conversation and told us about how child loss was handled at a Hanoi hospital in the early 1970s. At that time, she said, no one would consider bringing home a dead child from hospital:

> Everyone left them at the hospital. When I gave birth to my second child, they put him in an incubator and told me to go home. They said I could come back after five days to visit my child. When I came there was no child. They had not told me anything even though they did have my address. When I came they told me that my child died two days ago. I cried for a while, then I went home.

In spite of this discouraging initiation of her childbearing, Bà Xìn is now a successful mother and grandmother: her next three births resulted in three healthy sons, and today she is the central person within a large and flourishing family. In the eyes of Vân, therefore, she provided a model for how to handle reproductive disruption. Adopting the pragmatic and accepting stance to her loss that her mother-in-law advocated, Vân said, 'At first I intended to take it home, but then I thought again and realised that no matter what kind of funeral we arrange, the child is gone. Feeling sad does not solve any problem. This is something one has to overcome. This is the reason why I decided to leave it at the hospital'. Yet forgetting, she found, was not easy, but an act that required conscious effort:

> I try to forget. But when everyone else is at work and I am lying alone, there are moments when I can't help thinking and I feel so sad. So I have to call my friends and ask them to come and see me. I read books and newspapers, watch television, I do everything that helps me to think less about it. These are ways for me to try to forget. No matter how much I remember it, no matter how much I feel sad, it does not solve any problem. Whenever I see a child I think that I too have given birth, but I have no child, and I feel sad. But I must try to forget.

Most of the women we talked to described similar efforts to forget – and had similar trouble keeping away thoughts about their child. In this situation, Vân's mother-in-law supported her by encouraging her not to think too much and by assuring her of the necessity of the counter-mnemonic work she was undertaking. Like many other senior relatives we met, Bà Xìn sought to teach her daughter-in-law the necessity of striving to be carefree (*vô tư*) and cheerful (*vui*) in one's living and to avoid thoughts and speculations over sad events. She also ensured that her daughter-in-law did not get to see the foetus after abortion, fearing that the sight would leave a mental imprint on her mind that would never be erased. To capture such fears in words, people often used the term *ám ảnh,* a notion that describes situations where powerful memories of frightful events come unbidden, overwhelming and haunting people. Such intrusive and overwhelming re-experiences of the past – or 'traumatic flashbacks' – have also been described by U.S. Vietnam veterans and other people who have been exposed to violent experiences. Jonathan Shay describes the experiential power of such mental images: 'Once experiencing is under way, the survivor lacks authority to stop it or put it away. The helplessness associated with the original experience is replayed in the apparent helplessness to end or modify the reexperience once it has begun' (1994: 173). In a deliberate effort to protect the abortion-seeking women against being haunted by such powerful and intrusive mental images, health providers and relatives cooperated in ensuring that they were not confronted with the foetal body after the abortion: the dead foetus was instantly removed from the delivery room, and either health staff or relatives took care of its funeral.

After decades of warfare and extreme economic scarcity, it seems, people in Vietnam have developed an *ars memoria* (Kirmayer 1996: 191), an intentional and pragmatic forgetting of troubling events and searing experiences of loss. During our conversations about child loss and other reproductive disruptions, we encountered numerous examples of how this *ars memoria* was practiced and taught by elders to their younger relatives. Bà Cân's story provides one example of this. Bà Cân was eighty years old when we met her. She had lived her entire life as a farmer on the outskirts of Hanoi and had lost two of her nine children. Her second-born child, a boy, was nine months old when he became sick and died, and her next pregnancy ended in the birth of a stillborn girl. Bà Cân described in vivid detail her daughter's birth and death which took place about fifty-five years ago, and ended her story by saying: 'After the delivery the midwife said, "She is dead". They slapped her, but she did not cry. The midwife hugged me and said, "Sister Cân your child has died"'. When we asked her if she was seeking to remember or to forget this child, Bà Cân replied,

> Of course I had to try to forget her. But I could not forget her. But if I cried too passionately I would die. If I died, then who would take care

> of my children, my husband, my father, my mother? So my neighbour, an old woman, came to encourage me and she said, 'Little sister, do try to forget. Don't think about her, you are still young, you will have other children'. And so I had my next child, and he turned three and then four and he was walking around, talking, playing with other children, and so I did forget.

The death of Bà Cân's nine-month-old son a couple of years earlier had been even more painful for her:

> I had him for nine months, and he was a beautiful fair-skinned boy. At the time when he died he had just learnt to crawl. I had held him in my arms for nine months, I had breastfed him, and he was so dear to me. I tried to forget him, but I could not. At the time when I had my fourth child I was still missing him.

Bà Cân described her how her elders sought to make her forget this child by burying him at a site that she would not need to pass by in her daily life:

> They buried him behind the pagoda, there is a burial ground there. My father-in-law had him buried there so that he would be out of sight. We did not bring him home. He was only nine months old. He did not have bones, and he would reincarnate. So he was buried out of sight at that burial ground. There was a pagoda and a bamboo grove, and he was out of sight so I did not have to pass by him. Our family does not have land on that side of the pagoda. My father-in-law consoled me. He said, 'We must accept this, my child. I lost a son who was ten years old. He grew up to become a flower, and then a fruit, but he died. I wanted to die with him. But it is lucky you are still young, you can have many other children'. We still celebrate the death anniversary of his son who died. He has very strong spiritual power (*thiêng lắm*). When my husband and his brother were in the army, he followed them. So my father-in-law encouraged me and with time I felt better. My mother, my grandmother, my father-in-law – all encouraged me, and I talked to my husband, and with time I forgot and I did not feel so sad anymore.

As Bà Cân's story suggests, there is a long tradition in Vietnam of facilitating the 'forgetting' of painful and disruptive losses through practical actions and mutual emotional support. Remembering and forgetting, in this ethnographic context, are social practices that are firmly embedded in local worlds of intimate kinship ties and communal social lives; in the pragmatic actions that people undertake in order to shape their selves and lives in certain ways. Within everyday lives, people create 'landscapes of memory' (Kirmayer 1996) in which troubling and painful events are first socially acknowledged and then intentionally and collectively pushed out of social existence. While communal commemoration may, under some social circumstances, provide moral relief and emotional consolation (Kwon 2006; Layne 2003), the people we met in Hanoi insisted that sometimes collective forgetting is necessary in order to help individuals in pain to live and survive.

Conclusion

This chapter has shown that to comprehend people's responses to the painful loss of a child-to-be through a late-term abortion for foetal anomaly, we must consider not only local ontologies of human life and personhood, but also socially established strategies for moral and existential survival. Whereas in Euro-America, abortion is most often conceptualised through a Judeo-Christian framework where the foetus is seen as a symbol of life, innocence and nurturance (Ginsburg 1989), in an Asian country such as Vietnam, people make sense of early human life through engagements with Buddhist cosmology, spirit beliefs and the moral worlds of ancestor worship (cf. Sasson and Law 2009). These cultural traditions generate a wide interpretive space where different ontologies of foetal existence are mobilised, shaped through shifting situations, engagements and commitments.

It was within this complex realm that the women we met sought to come to terms with the moral ambiguities of their predicament. If Vietnamese ritual terrain is conceptualised as comprising a 'positive space' for ancestors and a 'negative space' for ghosts (Kwon 2006: 180; see also Feuchtwang 2003), then women and their relatives invented a third position for the foetus, one that defined it neither as a family member nor as a ghost, yet still asserted its humanity. By ritually 'remembering' the foetus, abortion-seeking women sought to maintain an identity as responsible mothers; ritual acts of incense burning and prayer were, in this context, moral gestures through which the women sought to (re)establish an identity as a good and caring mother by displaying maternal affection for the child they had lost. 'Forgetting', on the other hand, was a pragmatic strategy through which women, urged by their elders, sought to exorcise the foetal spirit from the family body in order to prevent it from causing future reproductive trouble. By first 'remembering' and then 'forgetting' the foetus, in other words, women sought to display maternal devotion to the child they had lost, while also de-linking it from the family body hoping, thereby, to enhance their chances of becoming mothers (again) in the future.

In sum, this ethnographic account suggests that while new biomedical interventions such as prenatal screening may place women and men across the world in novel and unprecedented dilemmas, such globalising technologies also engage in complex ways with already existing local efforts to ensure reproductive health and existential survival; efforts which unfold at the precarious and unstable intersections between life and death, where spirits, ghosts and mental phantoms thrive.

Notes

1. For decades, Vietnam has had one of the world's highest abortion rates. Under normal circumstances, the legal limit in Vietnam for pregnancy termination is twenty-four weeks of gestation, but if a foetal malformation is found there is no upper limit for abortion. Early abortions are affordable and easily available upon request at both public and private health service delivery points, whereas second- and third-trimester abortions are more costly and only performed by public providers at central or provincial level facilities.
2. Rayna Rapp's (1999) groundbreaking work on amniocentesis in New York City has been an important source of inspiration for the fieldwork I conducted in Vietnam. Another vital source of inspiration has been Lynn Morgan's work on foetal life and personhood (eg. Morgan 1998; Morgan 2002). I am grateful to Lynn Morgan for her generous comments on an earlier version of this chapter.
3. All personal names are given as pseudonyms.
4. The research explored the use of ultrasonography for the detection of foetal malformations and was conducted by a team of one Danish and ten Vietnamese researchers (for details on methodology, see Gammeltoft 2007a, 2007b). Our total sample included 55 women whose child-to-be was diagnosed through an ultrasound scanning as 'abnormal'. Of these women, 37 terminated the pregnancy while 18 carried it to term. This article is based on repeated interviews with the first 17 of the women who opted for abortion.
5. This urge to remember must be seen in the context of the strong moral expectations that surround death in Vietnam, where people are culturally and politically expected to remember and care for their dead (eg. Ho Tai 2001; Malarney 2002, 2003; Kwon 2006; DiGregorio and Salemink 2007; Jellema 2007).
6. If the body of the deceased is missing, the passage to 'the other world' is rendered difficult or impossible. Today, over thirty years after the

second Indochina War ended, relatives of soldiers missing in action are therefore still searching for their remains.

7. Classical Confucian tradition, writes Kwon (2006: 70), discourages commemoration of persons to whom the living do not owe ritual obligation.
8. People in Vietnam sometimes claim that a foetus or a neonate 'has no soul'. By this they seem to mean that it does not have a continued existence in 'the other world' along with family ancestors, but vanishes or reincarnates when it dies.
9. Until very recently, many young children in Vietnam did not survive their first days and months. If a woman experienced a series of miscarriages, stillbirths or neonatal losses, this would often be interpreted as an indication that the same (unviable) child kept being born to her, and elder relatives might mark its body (*đánh dấu*) with ink or another coloured substance in order to verify whether the next-born infant was indeed identical with this one.
10. In a few cases, people defined an anomalous foetus as a non-human being. One 76-year-old woman, for instance, claimed that the foetus that her granddaughter had carried was a 'monster' (*quái vật*). She was very upset when her granddaughter brought the foetus home and had it buried at the family's gravesite.
11. Of the seventeen women, seven brought the foetal body with them home while nine left it at the hospital (one abortion was performed in week fourteen, i.e., the abortion was performed through dilation and curettage rather than through induced delivery). Those who left the foetus at the hospital paid about US$30 to cover the expenses of the funeral rites, quite a large sum in a low-income country where a factory worker earned around US$60 per month at the time of our research.
12. In Confucian moral ideology, which underpins many kinship practices in Vietnam, only sons can perform ancestral rites and carry on the family line. Although kinship as practiced is considerably more complex than Confucian teachings suggest, Vietnam's increasingly skewed sex ratios suggest that cultural premium continues to be placed on male offspring (cf. Bélanger 2006).
13. As I discuss elsewhere (Gammeltoft n.d.), these ritual ambivalences seemed to also index partly repressed moral ambivalences about the abortion decision: while on the one hand asserting that they were sure that they had made the right choice, many women also expressed lingering doubts about whether the abortion had been justified (see Gammeltoft 2007b).

References

Bélanger, D. 2003. 'Indispensable sons: Negotiating Reproductive Desires in Vietnam', *Gender, Place and Culture* 13 (3): 251–265.

Bloch, M. and J. Parry. 1982. *Death and the Regeneration of Life*. Cambridge: Cambridge University Press.

Douglas, M. 1966. *Purity and Danger. An Analysis of the Concepts of Pollution and Taboo*. London: Routledge and Kegan Paul.

Feuchtwang, S. 2003. 'An Unsafe Distance', in C. Stafford (ed), *Living with Separation in China: Anthropological Accounts*. London: Routledge, pp. 85–112.

Gammeltoft, T. 2002. 'Between "Science" and "Superstition": Moral Perceptions of Induced Abortion Among Young Adults in Vietnam', *Culture, Medicine and Psychiatry* 26: 313–338.

———. 2007a. 'Sonography and Sociality. Obstetrical Ultrasound Imaging in Urban Vietnam', *Medical Anthropology Quarterly* 21 (2): 133–153.

———. 2007b. 'Prenatal Diagnosis in Postwar Vietnam: Power, Subjectivity and Citizenship', *American Anthropologist* 109 (1): 153–163.

———. n.d. 'Haunting Images. Prenatal Screening and the Politics of Choice', book manuscript in preparation.

Gammeltoft, T., Trần Minh Hằng, Nguyễn Thị Hiệp and Nguyễn Thị Thúy Hạnh, 2008. 'Late-Term Abortion for Foetal Anomaly: Vietnamese Women's Experiences', *Reproductive Health Matters* 16 (31 Supplement): 46–56.

Ginsburg, F. D. 1989. *Contested Lives: The Abortion Debate in an American Community*. Berkeley: University of California Press.

Hardacre, H. 1997. *Marketing the Menacing Fetus in Japan*. Berkeley: University of California Press.

Henshaw, S. K., S. Singh and T. Haas. 1999. 'The Incidence of Abortion Worldwide', *International Family Planning Perspectives* 25 (Supplement): S30–S38.

Hertz, R.1907 (1960). *Death and the Right Hand*. Aberdeen: Cohen & West.

Ho Tai, H. T. (ed.). 2001. *The Country of Memory. Remaking the Past in Late Socialist Vietnam*. Berkeley: University of California Press.

Huntington, R. and P. Metcalf. 1979. *Celebrations of Death. The Anthropology of Mortuary Ritual*. Cambridge: Cambridge University Press.

Jellema, K., 2007. 'Everywhere Incense Burning: Remembering Ancestors in *Đổi Mới* Vietnam', *Journal of Southeast Asian Studies* 38 (3): 467–492.

Kirmayer, L. J. 1996. 'Landscapes of Memory: Trauma, Narrative, and Dissociation', in P. Antze and M. Lambek (eds), *Tense Past. Cultural Essays in Trauma and Memory*. New York: Routledge, pp. 173–198.

Kwon, H. 2006. *After the Massacre. Commemoration and Consolation in My Lai and Ha My*. Berkeley: University of California Press.

LaFleur, W. R. 1992. *Liquid Life: Abortion and Buddhism in Japan*. New Jersey: Princeton University Press.

Layne, L. 2003. *Motherhood Lost. A Feminist Account of Pregnancy Loss in America*. New York: Routledge.

Malarney, S. 2002. *Culture, Ritual and Revolution in Vietnam*. Honolulu: University of Hawai'i Press.

———. 2003. 'The Fatherland Remembers Your Sacrifice. Commemorating War Dead in North Vietnam', in H.T. Ho Tai (ed.) *The Country of Memory. Remaking the Past in Late Socialist Vietnam.* Berkeley: University of California Press, pp. 46–76.

Morgan, Lynn M., 1998. 'Ambiguities Lost: Fashioning the Foetus into a Child in Ecuador and the United States', in N. Scheper-Hughes and C. Sargent (eds), *Small Wars. The Cultural Politics of Childhood.* Berkeley: University of California Press, pp. 58–74.

Morgan, L. M. 2002. ' "Properly Disposed of": A History of Embryo Disposal and the Changing Claims on Foetal Remains', *Medical Anthropology* 21: 247–274.

Moskowitz, M. L. 2001. *The Haunting Foetus. Abortion, Sexuality and the Spirit World in Taiwan.* Honolulu University of Hawai'i Press.

Oaks, L. 1994. 'Foetal Spirithood and Foetal Personhood. The Cultural Construction of Abortion in Japan', *Women's Studies International Forum* 17 (5): 511–523.

Oosterhoff, P., N. T. Anh, N. T. Hanh, P. N. Yen, P. Wright and A. Hardon. 2008. 'Holding the Line: Vietnamese Family Responses to Pregnancy and Child Desire when a Family Member has HIV', *Culture Health and Sexuality* 10 (4): 403–416.

Pashigian, M. 2002. 'Conceiving the Happy Family: Infertility and Marital Politics in Northern Vietnam', in M. Inhorn and F. Van Balen (eds), *Infertility around the Globe. New Thinking on Childlessness, Gender, and Reproductive Technologies.* Berkeley: University of California Press.

Pettus, A. 2003. *Between Sacrifice and Desire. National Identity and the Governing of Femininity in Vietnam.* New York: Routledge.

Phinney, H. 2005. 'Asking for a Child: The Refashioning of Reproductive Space in Post-War Northern Vietnam', *The Asia Pacific Journal of Anthropology* 6 (3): 215–230.

Rapp, R. 1999. *Testing Women, Testing the Foetus: The Social Impact of Amniocentesis in America.* New York: Routledge.

Salemink, O. and M. DiGregorio, 2007. 'Living with the Dead. The Politics of Ritual and Remembrance in Contemporary Vietnam', *Journal of Southeast Asian Studies* 38 (3): 433–440.

Sasson, V. R. and J. M. Law, 2009. *Imagining the Fetus. The Unborn in Myth, Religion, and Culture.* Oxford: Oxford University Press.

Shay, J. 1994. *Achillles in Vietnam. Combat Trauma and the Undoing of Character.* New York: MacMillan.

Stafford, C. 2003. *Living with Separation in China: Anthropological Accounts.* London: Routledge.

Chapter Four

VIOLENCE, POVERTY AND 'WEAKNESS'

INTERPERSONAL AND INSTITUTIONAL REASONS WHY BURMESE WOMEN ON THE THAI BORDER UTILISE ABORTION

Suzanne Belton

To develop policies or programmes that assist women and minimise unsafe abortions, we need to understand not only who the women are and their beliefs, but also how abortion takes place and who is practicing it, as well as the events that influence women's decisions to abort. This chapter explores why Burmese women on the Thai border utilise abortion. The majority of the women in this study are forced migrants, working in Thailand for a variety of reasons, including political and economic insecurity and to escape human rights abuses in Burma (Myanmar)[1]. It is based upon work completed for a larger study undertaken on reproductive health and the problem of spontaneous and induced abortion for this group of women (Belton 2005; Belton 2007). Despite the restrictive legal status of abortion in both Burma and Thailand, induced abortion using a variety of unsafe techniques remains an important means of fertility management among vulnerable Burmese women migrants (Belton and Whittaker 2007).

This chapter concentrates upon the experience of poverty and violence and their embodied form, 'weakness', among these women. Weakness appears here as an indicator for unsafe abortion. Violence and poverty, I argue, are common reasons for women to abort pregnancies.

The level of poverty experienced by some women on the border is shocking. One day a desperate woman came to the Mae Tao Clinic seeking help:

> Rose (my research assistant) is upset. She has spent the morning trying to explain to a woman that the Mae Tao Clinic will not purchase her eyes. 'She asked me how much for one eye. She said she had no money, no job and no place to live. She sold her mosquito net and clothes to buy food. She is hiding from the police. Her husband is ill and they are starving'. The desperate woman heard about the eye clinic and assumed they needed good eyes for people who had bad eyes. Her husband suggested the idea. He would sell one eye and she should sell one of hers. Rose gave her some money and a bowl of noodles but was still disturbed. The woman is five months pregnant. (S. Belton, fieldnotes)

For Burmese women, the competing tensions between paid work, family responsibilities, family size, relationship difficulties, domestic violence and sometimes rare unforeseen events are all implicated in the reasons to end pregnancy. The daily reality of poverty and suffering are the context for women's decisions. I will discuss these issues using a critical structural approach analysing abortion as resulting from the many forms of structural violence perpetuated against women in this region.

Context and Methods of the Study

Two main health facilities offer life-saving obstetric services to Burmese women with complicated abortions in Tak Province, located just inside the Thai border with Burma. One is the Burmese-led Mae Tao Clinic, the other is a Thai public hospital. Both of these facilities were approached for permission to access their medical case notes and to interview patients.

A research team composed of both male and female research assistants and led by myself conducted case note reviews and interviewed Burmese and Thai formally trained health workers, informally trained health workers, women admitted for post-abortion treatment, their partners, and abortionists. The site focused on the urban area and up to forty kilometres into the rural area away from the Thai–Burma border. A retrospective case note review of all women who attended the Mae Tao Clinic out-patient department in 2001 recalled 196 cases of early pregnancy loss and another thirty-six cases of serious abortion complications that were referred to the Thai public hospital. This was the first time that health data had been collected across nationalities and health systems: Thai, Burmese, formal and informal.[2] Despite abortion being a private and stigmatised topic, we found that both women and men were comfortable enough to discuss it if they were provided privacy and a respectful approach.

The limitation of this study was that it purposely sought women who experienced problems with terminating a pregnancy; only women who made contact with a health facility were included. There may have been other women who experienced miscarriage or abortion but who were not so incapacitated they needed to consult a health worker, or conversely were so ill that they were unable to contact a health worker.

The Mao Tao Clinic provides health services to the forced migrants from Burma who live and work on the margins of Thai society in Tak Province. The Clinic operates outside the formal Thai public health system but is tolerated by Thai authorities as it deals with thousands of cases of communicable diseases such as TB, malaria and HIV/AIDS, as well as offering maternal and child health care, family planning, immunisations, treatments for general illnesses and surgery and rehabilitation for trauma and landmine injuries (Maung 2004). The Mae Tao Clinic is a remarkable place, which also provides sanctuary to the resisters of the military dictatorship, the State Peace and Development Council, that rules the Union of Myanmar. The Clinic was established in 1989, after the democracy uprising and subsequent massacres in Rangoon (Yangon) and its continued operation is supported by funding from international Christian organisations and multiple philanthropic and foreign aid initiatives. The patients are all from Burma, either displaced by military aggression or economic desperation – refugees of one sort or another.

The law is a powerful structural element in enabling rights and accessing health care (Cook and Ngwena 2006). Abortion law in Burma is restrictive, only allowing a legal abortion if the woman's life is in danger (Ba-Thike 1997; United Nations Population Fund and Ministry of Immigration and Population Union of Myanmar 1999). Similarly, abortion is restricted in Thailand, although the medical regulations were recently modified (Whittaker 2004, see Nongluk Boonthai et al. this volume).[3] Although the majority of abortions in Thailand are technically illegal, terminations of pregnancy by medical staff in private clinics are available in Thailand. However, Burmese women are unlikely to use such clinics due to a lack of knowledge, prohibitive cost and inability to travel freely within Thailand.

Structural Violence along the Thai–Burmese Border

Paul Farmer and colleagues urge us to analyse the many forms of violence and oppression implicated in disease and health inequalities. They write:

> The adverse outcomes associated with structural violence – death, injury, illness, subjugation, stigmatisation, and even psychological terror – come to have their 'final common pathway' in the material. Structural violence is embodied as adverse events if what we study, as anthropologists, is the experience of people who live in poverty or are marginalized by racism, gender inequality, or a noxious mix of all of the above. The adverse events to be discussed here include epidemic disease, violations of human rights, and genocide. (2004: 308)

I argue that unsafe abortion is another such adverse outcome. Along the Thai–Burma border there is a long history of conflict, economic hardship, violation of human rights, discrimination, institutional neglect and individual abuse. Across the world the social gradients of morbidity and mortality from unwanted pregnancy are extreme; the poorest, the least educated and the most vulnerable die, or are maimed by perilous abortions performed by 'quacks', ill-trained or mercenary health workers who operate in environments that offer very few options to women (Grimes 2003; Rana, Pradhan et al. 2004; Singh 2006). These are material expressions of structural violence that work against women.

The structural violence which perpetuates unsafe abortion in the Tak Province may be analysed on three levels: systems, communities and interpersonal violence (de Bruyn 2003). In this chapter I interrogate the structural and institutional violence enforced on women from both the Burmese and Thai authorities, the communal values and expectations that allow gender-based violence to occur and support the continued utilisation of unsafe abortion, and the individual experience of violence. These multiple pressures are conflated in the reasons women and men give for abortions. I explore how this is embodied in the complaint of 'weakness' and how it operates as an indicator for unsafe abortion.

The Violence of the Burmese State: Why Women Move to Thailand

As events in 2007 confirm, the military regime in Burma is violent and oppressive towards Burmese citizens (Amnesty International 2006; Fink 2001; Global IDP Database 2007; Pinheiro 2007). Militarised societies are rarely conducive to civilian priorities. A large proportion of the Burmese economy is driven and directed by the military (Selth 1996). There are reports that education and health systems are underfunded and dysfunctional in Burma (Rotberg 1998; Back Pack Health Worker Team and Maung 2006). Skidmore (2003) discusses the extreme repression of civil society, the 'systematic violation of human rights' and the 'totalitarian utopia' in which the overt use of violence by the state is not the only means to control a population. She says, 'Violence is used selectively in "pacified" areas of Myanmar as a strategic tool of terror. The threat of political violence is what underpins and makes effective more subtle forms of control and coercion' (Skidmore 2003: 83). She also describes women's fear of rape and mothers' fears for their children. Fear is the element that controls the individual, ensuring both docility and compliance.

Petersen et al. (1998) document people arriving in refugee camps in Thailand, who have experienced and witnessed rape, forced labour, forced relocation, torture and murder in the course of their forced migration. Other authors investigating health or violence against Burmese women in Burma and in Thailand have recorded gross human rights abuses (Apple 1998; Beyrer 2001; Caouette and Pack 2002; Leiter 2004; Shan Human Rights Foundation and Shan Women's Action Network 2002). Skidmore writes, 'Violence against the Burmese population is perpetrated directly and indirectly, and this total disregard for the human rights and well-being of the population acts as a precursor for the flourishing of structured inequality, most especially among women and children, that pervades this avowedly equal and nonviolent country' (2003: 92). Mistimed and unwanted pregnancies are the inevitable outcomes of some of these experiences.

Belak (2002) describes human rights abuses such as sexual discrimination, rape, forced marriage and domestic violence within Burma and acknowledges the structural nature of discrimination faced by women living in Burma due to customary law, ineffective governance, conflict, forced migration, gender stereotypes and poverty. The women's stories in this text have a political purpose, which is to expose the violence of the regime and the impunity with which

Burmese women are ill-treated, either as ethnic minority women or forced migrants in Thailand or as Burmans living in a totalitarian state.

It is hardly surprising that thousands of Burmese move across the border to work in Thailand, a relatively peaceful country with employment opportunities. Cheap migrant labour is readily utilised in Thailand. Burmese women work in agriculture, manufacturing, service, tourism and construction industries (Pim Koetsawang 2001; Awataya Panam, et al. 2004; Leiter 2004). Many are employed without official work permits and can be easily exploited. Generally, Burmese employees in Thailand work for less money and have poorer working conditions than their Thai counterparts (Martin 2004). While some Thai employers are fair, many take advantage of the undocumented and vulnerable positions of their employees (Arnold and Hewison 2005). Attempts by Burmese workers to bargain for better conditions, or in some cases to simply be paid, are met with harsh retribution.

Female workers suffer discrimination in areas such as loss of privacy and restrictions to movement (Darunee Paisanpanichkul 2001). Living conditions in factories and on farms are poor. Female workers are scrutinised to ensure that they are not pregnant and are often dismissed if found to be pregnant. There is no right to maternity leave, or special conditions for women who need to do lighter duties or not have contact with noxious substances such as herbicides or pesticides in agriculture. This type of disregard for pregnant women is not confined only to Burmese women working in Thailand (Nongluk Boonthai and Suwanna Warakamin 2000) but I argue that Burmese women experience more discrimination.

Reasons to End a Pregnancy for Burmese Women

Burmese women, men and health workers give multiple and overlapping reasons why pregnancies are terminated. Health workers interviewed as part of our study were adamant that the family, community and socio-political situation are directly related to women's health status and are also the reasons why women choose to end their pregnancies. Naw Paw in the Out Patient Department of the Mae Tao Clinic listed some of these reasons:

> Poverty, difficult jobs, lack of knowledge about family planning; all influence abortion. People are unable to think well due to the politi-

> cal situation. Some husbands do not take care of their families, some women are abused and others just have many family problems. Some couples live together without marrying but they still get pregnant. Young women at school get pregnant and they have abortions. Sometimes the parents don't agree with the partner choice and if they are already pregnant and not married, this can be a cause of abortion.

Her colleague in the In-patient Department, O Htoo Kler, is also convinced she knows the motivations for abortion:

> I believe most Burmese people's economic situation is not good and that's the main reason why they abort the pregnancies. Others don't understand the consequences of abortion but some do. Some women really understand family planning but it is impossible for them to come to us due to security issues or other things that get in the way. Other women take *htou: zei* [Depo-Provera injection] but they don't follow the dates so they forget. Young women fall pregnant with their lovers due to inexperience. Some men have many wives, one in Burma and one here, and this causes problems. I remember one case where a mother came to me and she was three months pregnant and she told me the truth about inducing her abortion. Her second husband had sex with her daughter and she was now six months pregnant. She knew that it was too late for her daughter to have an abortion so she had one. She was very ill and I took her to hospital. I heard this story twice now – the other one was a husband who had sex with both sisters. These kind of men don't respect women at all!... Every time I see a woman with an abortion I get upset with the Burmese government. I directly blame them for reducing the economic standard so low.

The Burmese health worker summaries above are astute: during interviews women often talked about their motivation to end their pregnancy such as economic difficulties, relationship problems, a particular desired family size and mistimed pregnancy (See Table 4.1). The results of interviews with eighteen women who had ended their pregnancies found women often had multiple reasons.

The list may broadly be grouped into three categories: social and economic pressures; lack of contraceptive knowledge/ access or contraceptive failure; and relationship issues. The respondents in this study also spoke of persecution due to their political or religious beliefs or affiliation with particular ethnic groups. They told of their inability to feed their families, despite having paid employment, due to heavy taxation and rampant inflation. Many of the reasons given are the manifestations of the structurally and individually oppressive situation in which women find themselves.

TABLE 4.1 The reasons why Burmese women ended their pregnancy (n=18)

Theme Area	*Reason Given*	*Number of Women*
Problems with money and employment	Poverty, remittances and concern for children living in Burma	7
	Debts	2
	Unable to work if pregnancy continues/threatened by the boss	2
	No work/Not enough work	2
Problems with their relationship	Abuse and violence from husband	5
	Problems with husband, alcoholism, poor quality of relationship	3
	Abandoned by husband	2
	Widowed	1
Problems with contraception	No or incorrect knowledge of contraception	4
	Modern or traditional contraceptive accident	3
Problem with the number or timing of pregnancy	Wrong time, or does not want a child	3
	Too many children	1
	Pressured or advised to end the pregnancy by relatives/friends	2
Cultural belief	Bad luck to have this baby	1

Source: S. Belton, fieldnotes 2001–02

Poverty and employment pressures

Poverty and socioeconomic pressures were implicated in nearly every story of abortion. For example, a 24-year-old Burman woman with a history of four pregnancies presented with a miscarriage, itself the result of her vulnerable status as an undocumented migrant and fear of arrest:

> I have been pregnant four times now. I have had one induced abortion. This current problem happened because I had to run away from the police. We were in our house and the police were checking everyone and arresting our neighbours so I jumped off my house about one metre down to the ground. It had been raining, it was slippery and I landed directly on my bum. Not even one hour later I started to

> bleed and the baby came out. My placenta stayed inside and I bled a lot. I saw my baby, he was formed like a human... I am very sad. My parents were very sad as well. We all wanted this baby.

Further questioning revealed that her husband had secured a job in Thailand as a construction worker for seventy baht (US$1.60) per day and this was enough for her to decide that she could afford the current pregnancy. As she told us this story, she recalled her previous pregnancy and abortion:

> I stopped my last pregnancy when I was four months. [Tears well in her eyes.] I did it because my parents said that I had no job and my husband had no job. 'You will have many problems and why weren't you more careful?' ... I got married when I was eighteen. My first baby came when I was twenty and I have another one who is eighteen months. Then I decided to stop the next one. There was only two months between the next pregnancy. I don't want a baby too soon again.

Burmese workers in Thailand have very low and erratic incomes, well below what Thais consider normal. Women said that they had plans to work and save their money before having a child; some women had debts that needed to be repaid. A married woman with two children in Burma tearfully described her problems. Married for seven years, she had lived for one year in Thailand. She was ten weeks pregnant when she paid two hundred baht (US$4.60) for a stick abortion:

> The Thai boss is kind and helps us. He found out about the pregnancy and the abortion and he said, 'Why did you do that? We would look after you and your baby. You can leave it with us if you don't want it'. My boss took me to hospital and paid for the medicine. I will pay them back later. The Thai nurse and doctors said 'Calm down and tell us the truth'. They cleaned me up and afterwards the pain stopped. They told me that I did a bad thing. They don't understand why Burmese women do this. They will think that all Burmese women are bad women who kill their babies. When the pains came initially I didn't know what was happening. People talked about me in the factory and they gossiped and said that because I had so much pain that this was an induced abortion. I got a fever. My husband wants three children. I think we can have another one later in Burma but not now while we are trying to save money.

She was concerned that the Thai staff did not understand her reasons and that her husband did not support her decision to end the pregnancy. He had also told her to stop taking modern contraceptives because she had experienced side effects. She felt misunderstood and was aware that her behaviour could reflect on other women from Burma who live in Thailand. She had put her own children who are home in Burma and her husband's security before her own health.

While some women aborted without their husband's knowledge or consent, other women discussed their situation with their husband and they made the decision to abort the pregnancy together. A young husband spoke of his wife's stick abortion at four months:

> I knew she was pregnant. I feel unhappy because I don't have much money and I feel frustrated. I needed to borrow money to come to the Clinic. We are sad that we are so poor. In the last two months I sent my money to Burma. My wife was sick before the abortion with malaria – it comes and goes. She didn't take the medicine because she was afraid of it. So she got a high fever and got sicker. She couldn't walk for two months. I need to work to earn money. I think it is not the right time to have a baby. I want to have enough [money] behind me before I have a baby. It is expensive to look after a child. Women can't work in the factory after they have a baby, the boss doesn't like it.

In some farm and factory workplaces, the choice between pregnancy and paid work presents a dilemma. As most women who were interviewed did not have a work permit, they were a particularly vulnerable population. For Burmese women, Thailand does offer opportunities for economic advancement for families and individuals, and women were aware of this. Burmese men and women stated that they were saving for a better future by coming to earn money in Thailand and paying their debts. For some, pregnancy disrupted this plan.

Domestic violence: a direct and indirect cause of abortion

Violence against women is a common phenomenon. A multi-site study across ten countries conducted by the World Health Organization, found that violence against women was common, with 15 to 71 per cent of women (n=24,097) reporting physical and/ or sexual violence from intimate partners (Garcia-Moreno et al. 2006). There is little research on the violence women experience while they are pregnant and even less on women who have miscarried or intentionally aborted (de Bruyn 2003), but it seems that unwanted pregnancy and induced abortion are more frequent in women who experience domestic violence (Pallitto and Campbell 2005; Taft et al. 2004). One study (Kaye 2001) of 311 women seeking post-abortion care in Uganda (where abortion is illegal) found over half of the women disclosed surviving domestic violence and just under a quarter had had an induced abortion. Eleven per cent of women in the Ugandan study were targeted in the abdomen and about twenty-eight women said it was the reason they ended their pregnancy.

Many large-scale surveys of abortion fail to gather information about gender-based violence. Bankole, Singh and Haas (1998) for example, examined the data from twenty-seven countries asking why women have induced abortions, and noted that there were multiple reasons for not wanting the pregnancy.[4] The most commonly reported reason was to postpone or to stop childbearing and the next was socio-economic factors such as employment concerns or lack of support from the father. Partner relationship problems included the father not wanting the child and single motherhood, which in Asia was the reason for ending the pregnancy in between 1 to 14 per cent of cases. There is no explicit reference in the study to the characteristic of the relationships examined or of ongoing domestic violence, other than the statement, 'the husband or partner mistreated the woman because of her pregnancy' (1988:122) which seems to imply that the pregnancy caused the domestic violence. Rape and incest are not mentioned.[5]

A small number of foreign authors have begun to draw attention to the structural gender-based violence in Burma which flows across the border into Thailand. These researchers emphasise the connections between a totalitarian state and interpersonal violence (Belak 2002; Leiter 2004; Skidmore 2003). In this literature, themes emerge between women's status, their role in the family, individual rights versus family rights, women as property, and the construction of gender and sexuality. The authors reference the subordination of women within political and religious ideology, and the state and military's role in perpetuating patriarchy.

As seen in Table 4.1 in this study, abuse by the husband, being abandoned, or the poor quality of the relationship appears in several Burmese women's accounts of their motivation to end the pregnancy. Domestic violence is a relatively common experience for many women in Southeast Asia (Manderson and Bennett 2003), yet it is also highly sensitive. To elicit women's stories, questions were framed in the following way: 'How is your relationship with the father of your child(ren)?' and 'Do you ever feel scared of him?' These two questions elicited evidence of emotional and physical domestic violence. Five women out of forty-three reported surviving various forms of domestic violence ranging from emotional abuse to violent beatings. Violence may be the direct cause of some abortions and make other women feel that they do not want to form a family and be reliant on violent men. Domestic violence laws are not well articulated in Southeast Asia and even if they were, undocumented forced migrant Burmese women in Thailand cannot call on Thai police for protection.

The male research assistant interviewed ten men, five of whom were fathers of newborn babies. The other five had wives who had experienced a pregnancy loss. Three men out of these ten also disclosed their abuse of their wives. The abuse included beatings, assault while intoxicated, assault with weapons and verbal threats of murder. A Burman man married to a woman who had had an induced abortion said:

> We mainly quarrel at the end of the month before the salary comes. If I want to buy some alcohol she argues with me. Men spend more money. Sometimes I beat my wife but I do feel sad afterwards. My wife isn't afraid of me though, if she wants to say something she does.

A Shan man whose wife had just given birth said:

> I can always talk with my wife and we understand each other's ideas. We never have arguments. I am married for five years already. If she or I did something wrong we can tell each other and accept criticism. The only thing is when I get drunk she doesn't like it and she doesn't say anything – I think it scares her.

Another Burman man whose wife had terminated her pregnancy told the male research assistant he sometimes threatens her with a knife:

> We do quarrel sometimes and lately more than normal. About three times per month we have an argument. I think it is because of our economic situation. Sometimes I take a knife and show her but I don't touch her. I pretend but it is not real.

The Burmese and Thai health workers had not reported domestic violence in any of the medical records, but women were willing to talk about their relationships. The women confirmed what the men had said about their own controlling and threatening behaviour. A Karen woman who had had a miscarriage said:

> He doesn't respect me at all. My husband has had three wives in the past. He flirts around with older women all the time. He smokes,

> drinks and takes *ya ba* (amphetamines). When he is drunk he yells and swears at me and I am scared of him. I cannot say anything or speak back because I believe he will hit me. He hit me before so I know he will do it... I don't know how long I can stand this new husband! I am sad most of the time I am with him. He threatens me, 'I will kill you. I will throw you in the river'. I am very scared. He doesn't know about the miscarriage and I worry that if he knows he won't believe me and will take it out on me. I need to tell him carefully. I also worry about the debts we have.[6]

After running away from a forced teenage marriage, another Karen woman describes her second marriage:

> I am very scared of my husband. He is three years older than me. He always hits me. I think this is because I was married before. I have a daughter from this previous marriage. He doesn't accept that. We argue about this and about money. If we argue about money he hits me. His mother asks for money all the time but we don't have enough for ourselves. Then when I say this to him he gets angry and hits me and sometimes he gets a knife and tries to cut me. He hasn't cut me yet but he threatens me. One time he hit me with a plank of wood. There was a nail in the wood and it went into the skin on my back. He kicks me and punches me. I can't talk with him about my needs. If he doesn't like what I say he just hits me.

A Muslim woman told of inducing her own abortion with a bamboo stick:

> My husband always drinks and then he beats me. That's why I got rid of this baby. I don't want any more babies. Anytime he gets drunk he screams and shouts at me. I cannot say anything; if I did he would beat me. When he beats me I feel ashamed and cannot talk with people... I am scared of my husband... He scares me a lot. I worry when he is drunk and that he will hit me... I give up on husbands and I don't want any more babies. I want to look after the ones I've got already. The babies come too closely together. My husband has sex with me even when I tell him that I am bleeding. He doesn't listen to me. In Burma we all live in one house and sometimes I am too shy to have sex with my parents and the children around. He doesn't care. He is violent and loud. I really would like to leave him.

The case presented above was the only case we found of a woman inserting an object into her body by herself to induce abortion, as most informants asked a lay midwife for assistance.[7] Although we did not ask directly if women had experienced forced sex, this woman's account of not being able to decline sex when she menstruated or when she felt there was not enough privacy is important. Other women talked of their duty to please their husband or their fear of him finding another woman if they refused sex too often. This also implies some coercion in sexual relationships and an unequal power dynamic.

This Burman woman describes the physical violence she endures:

> I did this abortion because I have a lot of problems with my husband. I didn't mean to do it and in a way I would like the baby. My little girl is still small. I didn't experience so much pain and there wasn't so much blood loss. I can live with the idea of the abortion but I do understand that I have killed the baby. My heart is sad... I can't eat [tears come to her eyes and her voice is shaky]. People will probably talk about me but some will understand if they know my husband. My husband wants two children. At first I didn't let him know about all this but when I started to get sick I told him what I had done. He agreed with the abortion. I always feel that I have no rights to say anything and he decides everything. He hits me a lot. It hurts me. He kicks, punches and slaps me. I am always fearful of him. I have been married for four years.

She ended her twelve-week pregnancy with five sticks from the abortionist. In these cases domestic violence is an indirect and direct cause of the abortions. Women are unwilling to carry the baby or bond their relationship further with parenting.

I was grateful that these women were able to talk about their experience and I was surprised that men were also so candid about their behaviour. Clearly the husbands were aware of the methods they used to threaten and terrify their wives and they understood that it was a way to control them. It was not clear from these encounters whether the men also understood that their behaviour contributed to their wives' decision to end their pregnancies.

Weakness: the Embodiment of Distress

Clinically defined 'weakness', or distress, as experienced by these women can be a precursor to unsafe abortion in this context. Naw Paw, a senior medic in the Reproductive Health (RH) Out-Patient Department in Mae Tao Clinic, explained the diagnosis of weakness:

> The woman is dizzy, she has poor nutrition, she has cold hands and feet, she worries a lot. We do an examination. Sometimes there is anaemia but not always. We give her health education about nutri-

> tion, maybe multivitamins or ferrous sulphate. We say 'don't think so much' and we talk about meditation; something like counselling for her. A typical patient would be a woman who has had a lot of children, maybe more than four. She would come and say, 'Oh my goodness my period doesn't come, maybe I am pregnant again'. Also those who are breastfeeding they have weakness. The women who talk about food, family and money worries, they get weakness.

Weakness is a combination of physical, mental and social symptoms. Men do not get weakness in the same way that women do. Children never get weakness, except those that are poorly nourished. Skidmore (2002) describes *thwe aah neh* as a weakness of the blood, which can be classed as anaemia and can also be linked to irregular menstruation or amenorrhea. Many women who come to the out-patient department are measurably anaemic, but the health workers are detecting the socio-cultural determinants of weakness and not just the iron content of red corpuscles. Although the Mae Tao Clinic models itself on biomedicine largely informed by Western sources and also has many Western volunteers, the Burmese health workers use their own cultural diagnosis in interpreting their patients' symptoms.

Weakness is a common reason to seek out health care at the Mae Tao Clinic and is linked to poor reproductive health outcomes. The RH out-patient department's daily logbook records 167 visits during 2001 where women were diagnosed with weakness.[8] I first heard of weakness during interviews with forty-three women with post-abortion complications who were hospitalised and agreed to be interviewed. Three had a history of weakness in their medical records: a Burman woman in her ninth pregnancy who had had a spontaneous abortion, a Karen woman in her sixth pregnancy who had had two previous abortions in addition to her current induced abortion, and a Burman woman called Cho Cho (pseudonym) in her fourth pregnancy with three living children and in a violent relationship.

Cho Cho, age thirty-seven, had a medical history which included scabies and weakness. She had been pregnant four times and given birth to three children. She was employed on a farm in Thailand, which grew roses and vegetables. She lived, alongside hundreds of other Burmese migrant workers, in squalid conditions that deteriorated during the rainy season. She went to school for three years in Burma but could not read or write. She did not speak Thai despite living in Thailand for four years. She had neither a work permit nor a visa, which made her 'illegal', a non-citizen. She spoke very quietly and had an old scar over one eye that marked a past beating. She was still bleeding from the loss of the current pregnancy, possibly as a result of the most recent beating she had received from her husband:

> I feel very sad to lose this baby because I wanted it. When my husband started to kick me, I was lying in bed. I didn't feel very well at the time. Then he started to kick me. I don't think I will get back together with him... I fought with my husband. My husband kicked me in the back and stomach three or four times. My lower abdomen ached for two or three days. So I went to the massage woman. She only did gentle massage and I started to bleed two days after the massage.

This ambiguous statement may mean that she decided to end the pregnancy with a local abortionist with the oblique reference to the 'massage woman', or that the violent assault may have initiated the miscarriage. Her medical notes show that she received family planning counselling and contraceptive supplies two years prior to the current visit. She says she planned this pregnancy and wanted the baby but she suffers from *a: ne* (weakness) diagnosed by the Burmese health workers. She experiences violence at the interpersonal level from her abusive husband and experiences structural violence in the forms of grinding poverty and lack of life opportunities.

Weakness is a socially mediated expression of distress, when life has become unbearably hard and appears in psychosomatic forms. The medicalisation of social or cultural disruptions such as oppression, repression, violence and genocide is a widely accepted theme in anthropological and feminist writing (see for example Ginsburg and Rapp 1991; Kleinman 1995; Astbury et al. 2000; de Bruyn 2003; Petchesky 2003). The health workers at Mae Tao Clinic are perceptive clinicians who note the connections between the disease they are asked to treat, and the particular social circumstances of forced migrants living on the borders of both Thailand and Burma as citizens of neither country. Distress and suffering are invoked as warning signs by women that life has become unbearable in the illness of weakness; they are also given as reasons why pregnancies must be ended. Women talk not only of their own personal suffering but also the potential suffering of the unborn child and their living children, who may or may not be in Thailand with them.

Weakness as a diagnostic category is also found in India and Bangladesh and can be interpreted as an expression of distress (Kleinman 1995; Spiro 1967; Scheper-Hughes 1992). While narratives of weakness and white discharge are common, Ramasubban and Rishyasringa (2001) feel that weakness is more likely connected with a poor reproductive history and the combined stresses of poverty and gender-based violence. The authors note that the word 'weakness' (*ashaktapana*) in India combines physical and mental states. Women attribute the cause of their weakness (in order of frequency) to: excessive housework or caring for family members; tensions and stresses; sterilisation; burden of child bearing; erratic diet; neglect in childhood; neglect of diet during pregnancy; and poor postpartum care. Unemployment in the family, alcohol abuse and wife beating also play a role. Ramsubban and Rishyasringa (2001: 28) suggest that 'weakness' and poor reproductive health outcomes are related:

> Women who make the strongest association between problems during pregnancy and the onset of a chronic feeling of *ashaktapana* are those who have experienced spontaneous abortions, prenatal child loss, or delivered stillborn babies. Around half the women in this subgroup have experienced prenatal child loss or spontaneous abortions.

Similarly, in Bangladesh, Ross, Laston, Nahar and colleagues note that weakness (*durbalata*) is commonly mentioned in a country where, when a Bangladeshi woman 'reaches puberty, [she] has already experienced a lifetime of discrimination compared to males' (1998: 95). Among the women on the Burmese border, as in Bangladesh, weakness is both an indicator and cause of pregnancy loss.

Poor Contraceptive Knowledge and Access to Reproductive Health Services

Due to a lack of education and poor public health infrastructure in Burma, some couples are ignorant about the use of modern contraceptives. Many of the women interviewed were naïve about the specifics of sexual health and family planning. They were unsure about their menstrual cycles, fertility, and most modern contraceptive technologies. They relied on traditional herbal powders to regulate their menstruation and on market vendors to sell them products. The markets and pharmacies in Mae Sot contain a plethora of modern and traditional forms of fertility pharmacopoeia. The barriers to using contraception were knowledge, language, cost and the quality of the products, as well as the quality of information given by the vendor.

Unfortunately, even admission to hospital with post-abortion complications did not ensure that women were given access to family planning methods. The Thai public hospital staff were not able to offer any education or information to women and only required women to return to the hospital after six weeks for an out-patient visit. After any kind of pregnancy, it is possible to ovulate as little as two weeks later; this leaves women at the risk of further unwanted pregnancies.[9]

However, women were interested in understanding more about their contraceptive choices. Many women, at the end of their interview, asked about family planning methods, where to obtain contraceptives in Thailand, how much they cost and what we thought about them. The women in the Thai public hospital, who had the least access to this information, were especially curious and part of our finalising the interview was to offer women this vital information. But even if women understood how to control their fertility, their efforts were not always successful. Burmese men tended to see family planning as women's responsibility. Mae Tao Clinic runs a popular family planning clinic at very low cost to the client. Their records show low uptake on male methods of modern fertility control such as condoms and vasectomy. Very few male health workers were interested or assigned to work in this department. In many previous studies, Burmese men were willing to discuss contraception and sexual health although they held conservative views which perpetuate sexual double standards (Umemoto 1998; United Nations Population Fund (UNFPA) and Department of Health Union of Myanmar 1999; Caouette et al. 2000).

Conclusions

In this chapter, I have tried to draw together the many levels of structural violence experienced by Burmese forced migrant women, which are implicated in women ending their pregnancies. Structural violence takes multiple forms – from the historical and social forces that precipitate forced migration, to national levels of ineffective health systems and discriminatory employment laws. Poverty and problems with money and employment featured strongly in women's accounts of why they needed to abort. Women were overwhelmingly working wives who supported their families and paid debts. Women (and men) also disclosed domestic abuse and violence or problems such as alcoholism. In two cases pregnant women were abandoned by their partners and in one case the woman had been widowed. Burmese men hold a privileged position over women and can meet their sexual needs with relative impunity; generally men were not held accountable for unwanted pregnancies or abortions.

Most of the women I spoke with were barely literate and were naïve regarding modern contraceptive technologies. Their lack of access to basic and public health education were linked to their unwanted pregnancy. Lack of access to quality sexual and reproductive health services was a feature of women's experiences, even when admitted to hospital.

The literature on women's motivations to end a pregnancy generally derives from survey type research (Bankole, Singh et al. 1998; Bankole, Singh et al. 1999; Robotham, Lee-Jones, et al. 2005). Surveys need to be interpreted with caution, as prepared responses that offer only one category for answer simply do not reflect the complexity of lived experience and hence are limited in their ability to provide sensitive findings on issues such as the importance of violence and pregnancy terminations. Undesired fertility is not simply a personal problem where women commit violence against their own offspring because they are morally flawed, but rather has more to do with levels of violence that span time, place, culture, economics and politics.

Notes

1. In 1989 SLORC renamed Burma the Union of Myanmar (Myanmar Naing-Ngan), a transliteration from Burman. Burmese who resist the military regime interpret the use of the name as a political gesture supporting the regime. Throughout this chapter I use the term 'Burma' over the 'Union of Myanmar' because my exiled informants all referred to their country of birth as Burma when we spoke English together. I only use the name Union of Myanmar when quoting other authors or official sources such as the United Nations.
2. Demographic as well as biophysical and social information was collected. Quantitative data were analysed using basic descriptive statistics and qualitative data were analysed using thematic analysis. Preliminary results were fed back to practitioners and key community leaders at intervals to check for conceptual rigour in an iterative process (Liamputtong and Ezzy 2005).
3. Thai government regulations concerning abortion have recently been modified to allow for abortions to be performed in the following situations: '1. The pregnancy causes harm to a woman's physical or mental health. 2. The pregnancy is a result of rape. 3. The foetus is diagnosed with an anomaly or hereditary disease and the woman does not want

to continue her pregnancy'. In these circumstances abortions can now be performed without gestational limits at public hospitals, or at private clinics up to twelve weeks' gestation (Royal Thai Government Gazette 2005: 7 Book 22, Section 118g). See discussion in Boonthai et al. this volume.

4. Burma is not included in the twelve Asian countries surveyed but Thailand is included.
5. Most health workers are unable to detect domestic violence in their patients and rarely ask about rape or incest in their history taking; therefore it is not surprising that these experiences are not captured in the health sector data (Mazza et al. 1996; Hunt and Martin 2001).
6. *Ya ba* is 'crazy medicine' or methamphetamine. Amphetamines are manufactured in Burma and sold across the border into Thailand (Alford 2001; Yuwadee Tunyasiri 2001; Gutter 2001; United States Department of State 2003).
7. See Rozario and Samuel (2002) for more on self-induced abortions and lay midwives.
8. For comparison, other annual counts of the RH OPD logbook show abortion (196), STI/ PID (193), menstrual problems (110), urinary tract infection (76), and low fertility (46) as reasons for women to come to the clinic. I have excluded the numbers for antenatal care and family planning which exceed thousands of visits.
9. The Thai Public Hospital staff, Dr Cynthia Maung, Dr Bhensri Naemiratch and myself received a Safe Abortion Action Fund grant from the Planned Parenthood Federation U.K. in 2007 and have worked to improve many of these issues.

References

Alford, P. 2001. 'Burma boomtown that drugs built. A jungle hamlet grew into a city in a little more than a year', *The Weekend Australian*. Not dated, 12.

Amensty International. 2006. *Asia-Pacific Country Report Myanmar.* Retrieved 12 May 2007 from http://web.amnesty.org/report2006/mmr-summary-eng.

Apple, B. 1998. *School for Rape: The Burmese Military and Sexual Violence.* Bangkok: U.S. Office of Earthright.

Arnold, D. and K. Hewison. 2005. 'Exploitation in Global Supply Chains: Burmese Migrant Workers in Mae Sot, Thailand', *Journal of Contemporary Asia* 35 (3): 319–340.

Astbury, J., J. Atkinson, et al. 2000. 'The impact of domestic violence on individuals', *Medical Journal of Australia* 173: 427–431.

Awataya Panam, Khaing Mar Kyaw Zaw, et al. 2004. *Migrant Domestic Workers: From Burma to Thailand.* Salaya (Report): 227.

Back Pack Health Worker Team and C. Maung. 2006. *Chronic Emergency Health and Human Rights in Eastern Burma* (Report). Mae Sot, BPHWT Primary Health Care: 86.

Ba-Thike, K. 1997. 'Abortion: A Public Health Problem in Myanmar', *Reproductive Health Matters* 9: 94–100.

Bankole, A., S. Singh, et. al. 1998. 'Reasons Why Women Have Induced Abortions: Evidence from 27 Countries', *International Family Planning Perspectives* 24 (3): 117–127, 152.

———. 1999. 'Characteristics of Women Who Obtain Induced Abortion: A Worldwide Review', *International Family Planning Perspectives* 25 (2): 68–77.

Belak, B. 2002. *Gathering Strength: Women from Burma on their Rights.* Chiangmai: Images Asia.

Belton, S. 2005. 'Borders of Fertility: Unwanted Pregnancy and Fertility Management by Burmese Women in Thailand'. Ph.D. dissertation, Faculty of Medicine, School of Population Health, Key Centre for Women's Health in Society, University of Melbourne.

———. 2006. 'Post-abortion Care and Family Planning Theme: Sexual and Reproductive Health and the Millennium Development Goals in the Australian Aid program – the way forward'. *Submission to Parliamentary Group on Population and Development Roundtable discussion.* Retrieved 12 May 2009 from http://www.arha.org.au/

———. 2007. 'Borders of Fertility: Unplanned Pregnancy and Unsafe Abortion in Burmese Women Migrating to Thailand', *Health Care for Women International* 28 (4): 419–433.

Belton, S. and A. Whittaker (2007). 'Kathy Pan, Sticks and Pummelling: fertility regulation and unsafe abortion by Burmese women', *Social Science and Medicine* 65: 1512–1523.

Beyrer, C. 2001. 'Shan women and girls and the sex industry in Southeast Asia; political causes and human rights implications', *Social Science & Medicine* 53 (4): 543–550.

Caouette, T. et.al. 2000. *Sexuality, Reproductive Health and Violence: Experiences of Migrants from Burma in Thailand,* Salaya.

Centre for Reproductive Rights. 2003. *Breaking the Silence: The Global Gag Rules Impact on Unsafe Abortion.* New York.

Cook, R. J. and C. G. Ngwena. 2006. 'Women's access to health care: The legal framework', *International Journal of Gynaecology & Obstetrics* 94 (3): 216–225.

World Report on Women's Health 2006; Women's Right to Health and the Millennium Development Goals; Promoting Partnerships to Improve Access, 94 (3): 216–225.

Darunee Paisanpanichkul. 2001. 'Burmese Migrant Workers in Thailand: Policy and Protection', *Legal Issues on Burma Journal* 10: 39–50.

de Bruyn, M. 2003. *Violence, pregnancy and abortion: Issues of women's rights and public health: A review of world wide data and recommendations for action.* Chapel Hill, NC: Ipas.

Farmer, P., P. Bourgois, et al. 2004. 'An Anthropology of Structural Violence', *Current Anthropology* 45 (3): 305–325.

Fink, C. 2001. *Living Silence: Burma under Military Rule.* Bangkok: Zed Books.

Garcia-Moreno, C., H. A. Jansen, et al. 2006. 'Prevalence of intimate partner violence: findings from the WHO multi-country study on women's health and domestic violence', *The Lancet* 368 (9543): 1260–1269.

Ginsburg, F. and R. Rapp. 1991. 'The Politics of Reproduction', *Annual Review of Anthropology* 20: 311–343.

Global IDP Database. *Profile of Internal Displacement: Myanmar (Burma).* Retrieved 12 May 2007 from http://www.internal-displacement.org/8025708F004CE90B/(httpCountries)/59F29664D5E69CEF802570A7004BC9A0?opendocument&count=10000.

Grimes, D. A. 2003. 'Unsafe abortion: the silent scourge', *British Medical Bulletin* 67 (1): 99–113.

Gutter, P. 2001. 'Law and Money Laundering in Burma', *Legal Issues on Burma Journal* 10: 23–35.

Hunt, S. C. and A. M. Martin. 2001. *Pregnant Women Violent Men: What midwives need to know.* Oxford: Elsevier.

Images Asia. 1997. *Migrating with Hope: Burmese Women Working in the Sex Industry.* Chiangmai: Images Asia.

Kaye, D. 2001. 'Domestic violence among women seeking post-abortion care', *International Journal of Gynaecology and Obstetrics* 75: 323–325.

Kleinman, A. 1995. *Writing at the Margin: Discourse between Anthropology and Medicine.* Berkeley: University of California Press.

Leiter, K. 2004. *No Status: Migration, Trafficking and Exploitation of Women in Thailand, Health and HIV/AIDS Risks for Burmese and Hill Tribe Women and Girls.* Boston: Physicians for Human Rights.

Liamputtong, P. and D. Ezzy. 2005. *Qualitative Research Methods (Second Edition).* Oxford: Wiley-Blackwell.

Manderson, L. and L. R. Bennett, eds. 2003. *Violence Against Women in Asian Societies.* London: Routledge.

Maung, C. 2004. *Annual Report Mae Tao Clinic–2003.* Mae Sot.

Mazza, D., L. Dennerstein, et al. 1996. 'Physical, sexual and emotional violence against women: a general practice-based prevalence study', *The Medical Journal of Australia* 164 (1): 14–17.

Martin, P. 2004. *Thailand: Improving the Management of Foreign Workers.* Bangkok.

Boonthai, N. and Warakamin, S. 2000. *Induced Abortion: nationwide survey in Thailand.* Bangkok: ILO.

Pallitto, C. C. and J. C. Campbell. 2005. 'Is Intimate Partner Violence Associated with Unintended Pregnancy? A Review of the Literature', *Trauma, Violence, & Abuse.* 6 (3): 217–235.

Petchesky, R. P. 2003. *Global Prescriptions: Gendering Health and Human Rights.* London: Zed Books.

Petersen, H., J. Lykke, et al. 1998. 'Results of medical examination of refugees from Burma', *Danish Medical Bulletin* 45 (3): 313–316.

Pim Koetsawang. 2001. *In Search of Sunlight: Burmese Migrant Workers in Thailand.* Bangkok: Orchid Press.

Pinheiro, P. S. 2007. *Statement for the Fourth Session of the Human Rights Council.* Retrieved May 31 2009 from http://www.ibiblio.org/obl/docs4/2007-03-SRM-oral.pdf

Ramsubban, R. and B. Rishyasringa. 2001. 'Weakness [*Ashaktapana*] and Reproductive Health among Women in a Slum Population in Mumbai', in C. M. Obermeyer (ed), *Cultural Perspectives on Reproductive Health.* Oxford: Oxford University Press: 13–37.

Rana, A., N. Pradhan, et al. 2004. 'Induced septic abortion: A major factor in mortality and morbidity', *Journal of Obstetrics and Gynaecology Research.* 30 (1): 3–8.

Robotham, S., L. Lee-Jones, et al. 2005. 'Late Abortion: A Research Study of Women Undergoing Abortion Between 19 and 24 weeks Gestation', *Reproductive Health Matters* 13 (26): 163–164.

Ross, J. L., S. L. Laston, et al. 1998. 'Women's health priorities: cultural perspectives on illness in rural Bangladesh', *Health* 2 (1): 91–110.

Rotberg, R. I. 1998. *Burma: Prospects for a Democratic Future.* Cambridge: Netlibrary Inc.

Rozario, S. and G. Samuel, eds. 2002. *The Daughters of Hariti: Childbirth and female healers in South and Southeast Asia. Theory and Practice in Medical Anthropology and International Health.* London: Routledge.

Scheper-Hughes, N. 1992. *Death Without Weeping The Violence of Everyday Life in Brazil.* Berkeley: University of California Press.

Shan Human Rights Foundation and Shan Women's Action Network. 2002. *Licence to Rape: The Burmese military regime's use of sexual violence in the ongoing war in Shan State.* Chiangmai.

Selth, A. 1996. *Transforming the Tatmadaw: The Burmese Armed Forces since 1988,* Canberra: Strategic and Defence Studies Centre, Australian National University.

Singh, S. 2006. 'Hospital admissions resulting from unsafe abortion: estimates from 13 developing countries', *Lancet* 368 (9550): 1887–92.

Skidmore, M. 2002. 'Menstrual madness: Women's health and well-being in urban Burma', *Women & Health.* 35 (4): 81–99.

———. 2003. 'Behind Bamboo Fences: forms of violence against women in Myanmar' in L. Manderson and M.R. Bennett (eds), *Violence Against Women in Asian Societies.* London: Routledge, 76–92.

Spiro, M. E. 1967. *Burmese supernaturalism: a study in the explanation and reduction of suffering.* Englewood Cliffs: Prentice-Hall.

Taft, A. J., L. F. Watson, et al. 2004. 'Violence against young Australian women and association with reproductive events: a cross-sectional analysis of a national population sample', *Australian and New Zealand Journal of Public Health* 28 (4): 324–329.

Tamang, A. 1996. 'Induced Abortions and Subsequent Reproductive Behaviour Among Women in Urban Areas of Nepal', *Social Change* 26 (3–4): 271–285.

Thapar-Bjorkert, S., K. Morgan, et. al. 2006. 'Framing gendered identities: Local conflicts/global violence (Introduction)', *Women's Studies International Forum* 29 (5): 433–440.

Umemoto, N. 1998. *Like a Moth Chasing the Fire: An HIV/AIDS Audience Analysis of Urban Men in Myanmar With Recommendations for Strengthening HIV/AIDS Prevention Activities.* Rangoon: CARE Myanmar.

United Nations Population Fund and Ministry of Immigration and Population Union of Myanmar. 1999. *Fertility and Reproductive Health Survey 1997.* Yangon.

United Nations Population Fund (UNFPA) and Department of Health Union of Myanmar. 1999. *Reproductive Health Needs Assessment in Myanmar.* Bangkok.

Whittaker, A. 2004. *Abortion, Sin and the State in Thailand.* New York: Routledge.

Yuwadee Tunyasiri. 2001. 'No hopes for Burma's full cooperation against Wei: Thaksin says peace efforts may hinder drug baron's capture', *Bangkok Post.* Bangkok: 3.

Chapter Five

QUALITY OF CARE AND PREGNANCY TERMINATIONS FOR ADOLESCENT WOMEN IN URBAN SLUMS, BANGLADESH

Sabina Faiz Rashid

There is much disparity in the quality of abortion services, both in countries where abortion is legal and where it is illegal. There is no guarantee that, just because the service is permitted by the state, it will be safe (Warriner and Shah, 2006; Standing, 2007). Abortion in Bangladesh is legally restricted under the Bangladesh Penal Code. However, menstrual regulation (MR), which is defined as a method of ensuring/confirming non-pregnancy for a woman at risk of being pregnant, is allowed.[1] The World Health Organization (WHO) defines menstrual regulation as 'early uterine evacuation without laboratory or ultrasound confirmation of pregnancy for women who report delayed menses' (WHO 2003: 22). MR services up to ten weeks of pregnancy are legally available at all major government hospitals and health facilities, as well as being provided by local NGOs and private clinics. Despite the legality of MR services, a report by Akhter (2005) estimated that there are over 400,000–500,000 clandestine abortion service providers in Bangladesh, including traditional practitioners and medical personnel who have no formal training. In Bangladesh, as will be apparent in this chapter, the term 'MR' is used more broadly by professionals and lay people to refer to a broad range of procedures. 'MR' services provided to women include abortions performed on women in middle and late gestations, long after the ten-week limit. Abortion studies remain scarce, with almost a complete absence of research on the quality of MR services, particularly the role of the private sector where many clandestine providers operate and remain unmonitored, resulting in potentially risky experiences for poor young women.

This chapter is based on ethnographic research conducted among married adolescent women between 2001–2003 in Phulbari slum in Dhaka. These women shared the realities of their lives, their reasons for pregnancy terminations, and their experiences in accessing MR services against a backdrop of lesser choices and an unregulated private health sector in the urban environment. A number of methods were utilised by myself and my research assistant including a survey of 153 married adolescent women, fifty follow-up in-depth interviews, and eight case studies of women and their families; in-depth interviews with key informants, community members/leaders; and interviews with informal and formal health providers from the community.[2] I highlight here how structural and social inequalities come together to shape decision-making surrounding pregnancy terminations (see also Belton, this volume).

For poor young women living in slums in Dhaka city, the effects of growing urban poverty and migration have brought with it shifting gender and power relations, unemployment, and unstable family life, which result in greater vulnerability and risky reproductive experiences for many of them. Insecurity, financial constraints, household politics, marital instability, and other social pressures compel married adolescent women to end their pregnancies. Despite the government services available, many young women seek cheaper abortion methods or access terminations from NGO clinics or dubious private-sector facilities, which may be unsafe. When young women do seek legal MR services, the economic considerations of the health providers themselves overshadow the quality of care available to women: NGO health workers form part of an informal referral network in which they serve as brokers for private clinics and compete with one another to find potential clients. Providers in private clinics with unknown qualifications and capabilities promise NGO health workers cash in exchange for clients. This results in unsatisfying levels of care as well as potentially risky services.[3] In contrast, the local NGO clinic in the slum provides safe MR services within the legally accepted period of eight to ten weeks of pregnancy, but poor after-care and the insensitivity of providers leave young women vulnerable. Adolescent women's MR experiences at both NGO and private facilities demonstrate that quality care, access to information, and gender-sensitive support for young women remain crucial yet neglected areas in abortion provision.

This chapter is divided into three main parts. The first part briefly surveys the situation of adolescent within Bangladesh's increasing urbanisation, and then I go on to discuss young women's reasons for abortion; the next section explores the experience of pregnancy terminations in the private clinics and in the local NGO clinic. In the final section, I explore the implications of my findings.

Background: Adolescents and Urbanisation

As a group, adolescents are of special interest in Bangladesh because they constitute more than 22 per cent of the population; thirteen million adolescents are girls and fourteen million are boys (Nahar et al. 1999). The 1999/2000 Bangladesh Demographic and Health Survey (BDHS) found a median marriage age among all women aged between fifteen to forty-nine (including both married and unmarried women) of 14.7 years. The importance placed on fertility for newly married adolescent girls results in high birth rates and low rates of contraceptive use. The current fertility rate of those young women aged between fifteen and nineteen years old is 147 per 1,000, ranging from 155 in rural areas to 88 in urban areas. This is the highest fertility rate for this age group in the world. In addition, poor married adolescent girls are less likely to use any method of contraception than the national average: 30 per cent compared to the national figure of 49 per cent for all women (Arifeen and Mookherjee 1995). Bangladesh also has one of the highest maternal mortality rates in the world, estimated to be 320 per 100,000 live births (GoB–UN 2005). One consequence of early marriage and childbearing is a higher death rate among adolescent girls than boys aged fifteen to nineteen: 1.81 compared to 1.55 per 1,000 (BBS 1997).

Compared to their rural counterparts, married adolescent women in the urban environment are particularly vulnerable because of their age, gender and poverty. With continued urban growth fuelled by the influx of the less educated and the very poor who have lost their livelihoods in their native villages, cities in Bangladesh have become the location of some of the worst poverty, with burgeoning slum settlements often juxtaposed against extreme wealth (Caldwell et al., 2000). It is argued that, although in the past urban populations could expect much lower levels of mortality and morbidity than their rural counterparts, urban rates can be as high as rural rates and are often higher, especially among the poorest of this population (Caldwell et al. 2000; see Perry 2000).

There are now 9,048 slums identified in six cities in Bangladesh (Islam et al., 2006). Urban slum dwellers as a population are particularly visible, as they are most obviously impoverished. By 2015, the population of Dhaka city is projected to double to an estimated twenty-one million because of the rapid growth of rural-to-urban migration (Perry 2000). Forty to 70 per cent of Dhaka's urban population growth is now attributed to rural to urban migration (Islam et al., 1997; Afsar 2000). Urban slum dwellers constitute 30 per cent of the total fourteen million population of Dhaka (2002). Unable to find affordable housing, many arriving migrants and the poorest residents in the city live in insecure tenure, setting up or renting small rooms in shacks with mud floors and bamboo or tin/polythene roofs in settlements built on vacant or disused land, never knowing when their settlements might be demolished (Islam 1996).[4] High population densities and an absence of latrines, sewage and drainage facilities, as well as inadequate water and electricity supplies, characterise slum neighbourhoods. It is reported that almost 60 per cent of the urban poor live in extreme poverty, and the remain-

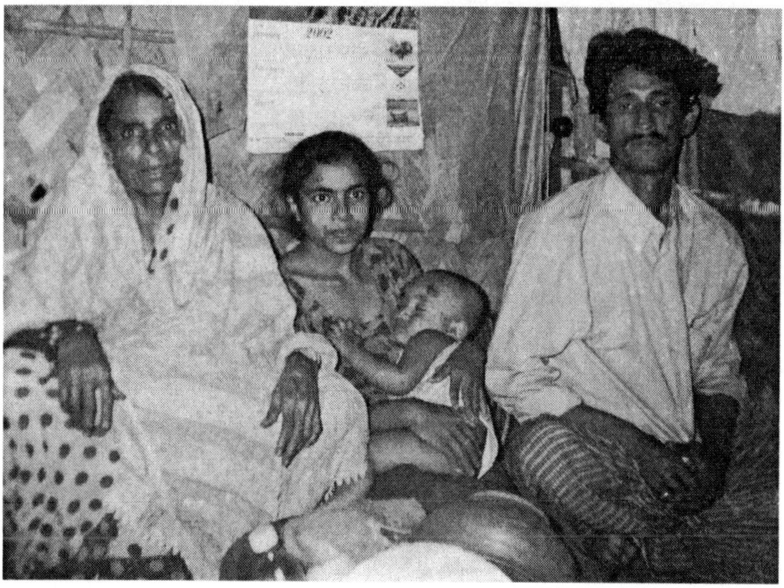

ILLUSTRATION 5.1 A family waiting to be evicted from Phulbari slum (Photograph: S. Rashid).

der in 'hard core' poverty, in which families survive on a monthly household income (1995) of only US$44.00 (Islam et al., 1997).[5]

Established in the early 1980s, Phulbari slum saw its residents evicted by the government in 1993, but the same residents managed to regain control of the area within a short period of time. They were once again evicted in July 2002, and have not been able to reclaim their space, as of May 2006. New buildings are being developed in the area and the entire land has been cordoned off.[6] We tracked the case study subjects by spending time near the evicted slum, visiting the health providers who had relocated their clinic nearby, talking to other women and men who spent the first few weeks hanging around the neighbourhood, who assisted us in locating our respondents.

Reasons for Pregnancy Terminations

Of the 153 women interviewed, twenty-seven reported that they had terminated a pregnancy, of which eleven adolescent women felt compelled to end their first pregnancy against their own wishes. A number of reasons were given for ending the pregnancy, such as poverty and financial constraints; being 'too young and not ready to have a baby', 'already having a young baby/child', 'shame'; marital instability; the family or husband's opposition to the pregnancy; and job insecurity. Below are some narratives in which married adolescent women describe their reasons:

> *Shohagi:* Look, I didn't want any more children because we are poor and my in-laws are very poor. Every day we have to give one hundred and fifty Taka to my in-laws. I have already one child [girl]. He [husband] earns but he is the sole income earner for the family. He is the only son. Reza said to me, 'Look, we don't need any more children,' and I agree with him, so we decided not to keep this baby.

Shohagi's case illustrates the most commonly cited reason among adolescent women: poverty constraints and the pressure of already bringing up one child were often mentioned in the slum as reasons for ending a pregnancy.

Marital instability was another repeatedly mentioned concern for many young women in the slum. Slum environments allow for a certain degree of anonymity, as men and women can easily relocate to another slum in the city without fear of social sanctions, which they would face in the tighter knit village communities, a finding reported elsewhere (Jesmin and Salway 2000). Of the 153 young women interviewed, twenty-four were already separated or had been abandoned by their husbands or were in their second marriages. Four women were sharing their husbands with a co-wife and another three suspected their husbands of having another woman or co-wife.[7]

In Beauty's case, her husband was always disappearing and there were rumours that her husband had remarried. She stated:

> Before, I was five months pregnant and I got rid of the child. This is because if I am not going to do household with him [live with him] then why should I keep his child? I went with my sister to a private clinic in Mirpur ... My husband heard later on that I had got rid of the child and asked me, 'Why did you get rid of my child? The child is mine'. Then I said, 'In my life I have no need of you so I also have no need of keeping your child either'.

Beauty's case was unusual because she decided not to go ahead with the pregnancy as she did not want to risk raising a baby on her own. Her courage came from strong natal support from her mother and sisters, who also lived in the slum nearby.

Micro-level politics in the household forced Parveen to end her pregnancy. She had eloped with her husband. Her husband did not work properly and they were dependent on her husband's parents and brother-in-law to manage their household. Her in-laws were not supportive of her pregnancy and had not accepted the marriage and were not willing to support her.

> *Parveen:* The first time I fell pregnant, I aborted the baby. My husband asked me to get rid of the child. The sole reason was that then there was a lot of poverty and financial constraints, so I had to abort. Also, beyond this, my older brother-in-law's wife was pregnant. My husband did not work properly and they [in-laws/brother in-law] were not ready to support my baby and me. So we decided not to have the baby, so I could continue to work.

Soon after the termination of the pregnancy, her husband abandoned her and Parveen was forced to move back to her father's household again and she started working.

With growing urbanisation there are many young women working outside the home, mainly in garment factories. This involves working alongside male strangers. Seeking termination of pregnancies can lead to accusations and rumors of infidelity from community members and even from husbands. Thus, women who seek

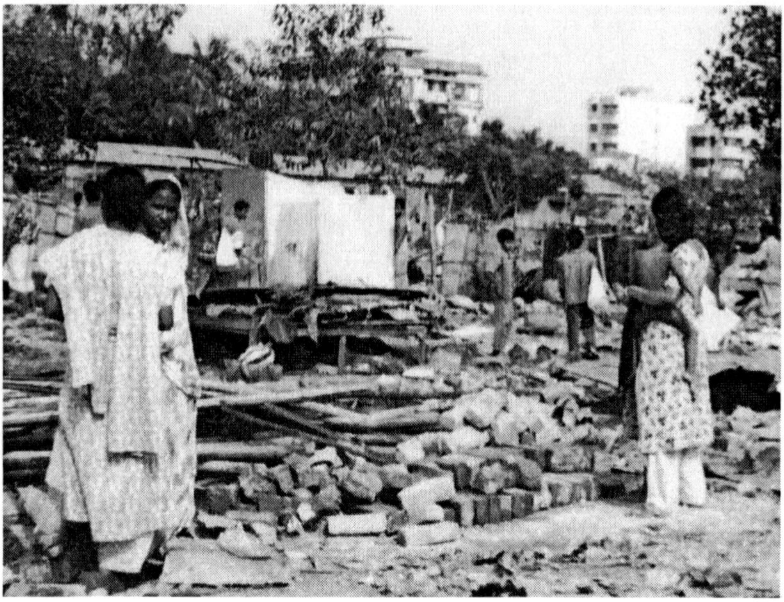

ILLUSTRATION 5.2 Residents watch one section of Phulbari slum being demolished, Dhaka, July 25, 2002 (Photograph: S. Rashid).

abortion or MR can experience gendered stigma from within the family and wider community.

As these case stories highlight many young women are powerless and vulnerable. Given their situation and general marital instability aggravated by urban poverty, their negotiating power is minimal, and in some cases, the ability to earn an income is given priority over having a baby. Eleven young women reported that they felt compelled to end their pregnancies because of power relations and politics in the household. With a lack of acceptance from in-laws, or husbands not ready to provide support, some young women were expected to continue working to provide an income to the household and hence were forced to abort their pregnancies.

In other cases, young women spoke of the shame of having a baby too soon, or justified the pregnancy termination on moral grounds. In Rosina's case, both of she and her husband were embarrassed about the pregnancy, which was perceived to happen 'too soon after marriage'.

> *Rosina:* About five or six months ago, I became pregnant. My husband asked me to get rid of the child. This is because my husband said, 'What will people say if we have a child now?' This was very embar-

> rassing for him. 'My friends and my own uncles have not got married as yet. Now if I have a child this is a big shame for me'. My mother-in-law and I didn't want to abort the child, my husband wanted me to get rid of the child.

This was mentioned by another young couple who also chose to terminate the first pregnancy, citing similar reasons of 'shame' and being too young to have a baby so soon after marriage. As Rosina explained: 'What will people say? We just got married a few months ago... people will talk'. Another woman, Purobi explained: 'It is sinful to end a pregnancy but is it not more sinful to have a baby but then not be able to breast-feed it properly, or be unable to feed it properly because we have no money?' A few of the young women also suggested that it was 'acceptable to end the pregnancy before three months as the baby was not fully formed then'. Similar understandings were found among local healers (who provided various methods for inducing abortions) and even among health providers.

Pregnancy Terminations

Women terminated their pregnancies either through legal menstrual regulation, or through illegal means, which is sometimes the first preferred option, as it is much cheaper.[8] Of the twenty-seven young women who had terminated a pregnancy, thirteen reported that they had sought menstrual regulation services and fourteen attempted unsafe means to terminate their pregnancies. As Akhter (2000) reports, induced abortion constitutes one of the major causes of maternal mortality and morbidity in the country.[9]

Termination methods ranged from using herbal pills, insertion of roots, liquid drinks purchased from local healers, and the consumption of packets of birth control pills from the pharmacy and local slum clinic. For example, Seema, Bina and Moni, (all married adolescent women) reported ingesting local drinks made by the local *kabiraj* (local healer), but when that didn't work they resorted to menstrual regulation services from the local providers working in the NGO clinic inside the slum. The cost of a menstrual regulation at the local NGO is approximately Taka 350 (US$5.00), which does not include the costs of medicine or transport to the clinic. This may explain the preference for cheaper options described above which cost from Taka 50 to 70 (US$1.00). Although government clinics officially claim to provide free procedures, in reality, women have to pay from Taka 30 to as high as Taka 550, (US$0.75 – $13.75) with the average amount spent Taka 290 (US$7.25) (Hossain et al., 1997). Moreover, in a number of cases observed, adolescent women were rejected from receiving MR services from the local NGO clinic in the slum as they were pregnant beyond the eligible period of time (8–10 weeks) to receive an MR.[10]

A number of factors shape the delay in accessing timely MR services; in some cases young women in the slums are married as young as thirteen or fourteen years of age and did not realise they were pregnant by the time they accessed services from the clinics and were rejected for coming beyond the safe period of termination of eight to ten weeks. In other cases, young women could not convince their husbands to let them keep the baby or were pressured by other social and economic factors much later, which delayed the process of seeking timely services. Other young women and their families opted for cheaper options from local healers given the shortage of cash available and only accessed formal services when these methods did not work. These delays caused by age, unequal gender and power relations, and poverty places young women's lives at considerable risk. The rejection meant that young women needed to find another provider as soon as possible, preferably a private health provider who would be willing to terminate the pregnancy, leaving them vulnerable to risky terminations from clandestine clinics and staff operating in the city without a license and with dubious qualifications.

Providers: the racket of referrals

Daily observations at the local well-known NGO clinic set up inside the slum found a regular stream of adolescent women as well as middle-aged women seeking pregnancy terminations. The clinic provided MR services at its headquarters, located thirty minutes away by car. To avail themselves of MR services, women had to firstly undergo a urine test confirming the pregnancy and gestation. Young women were then taken to the main office by a health provider to have the procedure. Women are expected to cover the costs of transportation, Taka 30, plus the costs of the termination itself.

Observations also found that young women seeking pregnancy terminations were normally questioned upon entering the clinic, with the three health workers competing to retain clients and take them to private facilities with which they maintained referral linkages. Health workers also relied on their own informal network of relations within the community to find young and older women who were seeking information on MR services. The incentive for the health staff working at the NGO clinic to take poor women to potentially dubious private clinics is that they are paid a sizeable amount, earning close to Taka 100–150 (US$1.40–2.15) per client, a substantial amount of money for poor health workers and their families. In contrast, they only earn a fixed amount of Taka 50 (US$0.71) from their local NGO clinic. If a pregnancy goes beyond the safe period of eight to ten weeks, the cost of termination increases, resulting in health workers receiving higher commissions.

A large priority for the health workers, who remain underpaid and only earn Taka 1,300 per month (US$18.50), was to gather and refer as many clients as possible as there was a large amount of money to be earned from MR services from private clinics. One of the workers bluntly said, 'I try and do MR for the women here (private clinics) and that is how I earn money – otherwise it is not possible for me to survive on my income. I have three children to feed and no husband to support me'. One of these health workers also sold Indian saris (popular in the slum) part-time in the afternoons to supplement her income. The saris cost from Taka 200–250 (US$3.00–4.00). She said, 'When I go to the office I take the cloth and saris in the bag and then [when she does field visits or after she is done] I sell the saris and cloths'. The competition for getting clients and taking them to a private clinic is so fierce that we found fights and arguments taking place between the providers. One day we observed one of the health providers in a bad mood, complaining, 'She took all three patients [MR patients] today, she will earn a lot of money ... she didn't even leave one for me'. Another health worker pointed out, 'If I had more money I could do my own MRs and earn more money. We don't need a doctor to do this procedure. I could do this on my own...'

It is also unclear whether staff who work in these particular private clinics are qualified or trained to carry out MR procedures. The health workers stated that the private practitioners used vacuum aspiration to conduct the procedures and therefore it was safe. They did not seem to be concerned about whether the people providing services in these clinics were trained or qualified to do so, even if a pregnancy was beyond the safe period of eight to ten weeks. The health workers were very familiar with two private facilities and routinely took the young women and older women there.

MR services at the private clinic

After much pleading, we managed to convince one NGO health worker to allow us to accompany her and her client to one of the private clinics to which she takes her clients. We were requested not to ask any questions. The clinic which is located ten minutes away from the slum, had no sign post outside indicating its services, but there was a dingy staircase with the tiny clinic located on the second floor of the building. The owner peered suspiciously at us and after some discussion with the health worker, allowed my research assistant and me to enter the reception area. We waited on one of the benches and overheard the following interaction between a young woman and the provider at the clinic:

> *Provider:* How many months pregnant are you?
>
> *Girl:* Three months pregnant.
>
> *Provider:* How much money have you brought?
>
> *Girl:* I have brought 250 Taka [US$3.50].
>
> *Provider (angrily):* I won't do it with this amount of money. Go to your NGO clinic. This is my business; I cannot do it for less.
>
> *NGO worker (pleading on the girl's behalf):* She is a poor person – please do it… If they could give more money wouldn't they give you more?
>
> *Provider:* I can't do this – this is my business. Please go elsewhere – go to the local NGO clinic.
>
> *NGO worker:* Sister, they are poor people, do it for them. If they had more money wouldn't they give it to you?
>
> *Provider (looks to me):* They always bring the very poor women to me. What can I do? I get so angry! I scream and shout but I do it…

Further discussions took place quietly between the NGO worker and the private provider and they reached an agreement about payment. A little while later, the private provider took the girl inside the room for MR. After about twenty minutes, the girl came outside the room, wincing in pain and she was made to lie down in a narrow room, right next to the waiting area. She kept sobbing quietly. The NGO health worker became restless to leave and said to the girl, 'Are you done with your rest? Let's go home now'. The girl walked the ten minute distance back to the slum with the health provider. As the NGO worker entered the slum, she turned to me and said, 'Don't ever tell anyone that I didn't go to our local NGO clinic … you see, this month I only got this one patient – I haven't done a single MR this month. What am I to do?'

There appears to be no counselling regarding young women's health concerns about menstrual regulation and rarely any follow-up care of patients after the procedure takes place. Critically, there was no information given on family methods thus missing an opportunity to provide young women with information which reduces the possibility of women having to seek repeated terminations. In addition, the lack of support from the local health provider on way to the clinic and after the procedure meant that young women suffering from feelings of fear, sadness and guilt, coped on their own with little emotional support.

Young women spoke of not knowing what to expect and of experiencing extreme pain and trauma after the MR experience. One young girl shared her story, which reflected the typical experience for many. She said:

> *Apa* [sister], I don't know about others but I can definitely tell you about my experience. I had never done wash [MR] in my life. I was very scared when I went to do the MR and no one explained anything to me. I have heard from others if you do wash then you don't feel much hurt – sometimes you don't even realise and it is over. *Apa*, but I had so much suffering I don't think I can even explain the kind of pain I went through. I had a lot of pain. It felt like my liver and heart were being ripped out of me. They didn't just put the '*nor*' [vacuum aspirator] in once but three times they put it inside me. I don't know how people say that they have had two to three washes (MR)... I can't imagine going through this again. I lost consciousness. I was so scared and the intense pain – I just lost my senses.

Another adolescent woman said, '*Apa,* no one tells that it is much more painful than childbirth!'

While quality of care is not very good in NGO and government clinics, if the MR is incomplete, the clinics do the procedure again for free, whereas private facilities do not do a repeat procedure for free. More dangerously, unlike the local NGO clinic in the slum where fieldwork was conducted, the private clinics were willing to provide MR services beyond the safe period. An NGO worker reported the dilemmas of conducting an MR with a woman beyond a certain point as the costs are much higher. She explained:

> The woman next door – she has four children and now she is five months pregnant. She didn't even know she was pregnant. Now she wants to get rid of the child. She can't keep the child. I have told Auntie [private provider] who asked her to bring Taka 1000. As it is at the five months stage, there is much more risk so therefore the higher costs. The woman wanted to give 800 Taka but Auntie said that it is not possible to do for 800 Taka; 1000 Taka, is the cost, and she will only do it at that price.

Although health workers want to ensure their commission, they also experience social and emotional stress if there are MR related complications from a private clinic, as there is no one else accountable except the provider herself, leaving her vulnerable to social ostracism or worse. In contrast, if there are problems or complications as a result of an MR in an NGO, the health provider can always refer the client and client's family to senior staff at the local NGO (see Seema's case below). A health worker shared her terrifying experience when the client, who was almost five months pregnant, passed out after an MR in a private clinic:

> *Apa,* you won't believe what happened to me today… it was awful… Mortoza's wife was okay when I brought her back but as soon as we entered the slum, she suddenly became senseless. My heart stopped beating, I was so scared. So then everyone [in the health worker's household] started running around. We made her lie down in my niece's room. I poured cold water on her head and fed her warm milk and then she became better. We warmed up oil and I wiped it on the legs and hands and feet. My brother-in-law massaged her. If anything happened to her then I would be in jail. I was so scared but she was okay after lying down for some time. Much later, we informed her husband who came and brought his wife home. We told him to feed his wife spinach and eggs – I also bought some medicines for her…

Some of the married adolescent women pointed out that unmarried, separated and widowed women who preferred to do an MR in secret were completely dependent on informal providers who would decide where to go for the termination. As private clinics/facilities actively recruit brokers (pay health providers) for referrals, young women who remain uninformed are at risk of poor care at these facilities. There is a wide range of easily accessible pharmacies and small private clinics in the city providing services, with most remaining unregulated and many staffed by untrained and unqualified people. For example, in one case, a young woman went to the local clinic provider who promptly took her to a private clinic near the slum to avoid being seen by others in the slum. The NGO health worker explained the woman's predicament:

> She lives in slum number two and she only got married about two months ago. She lives next door to Rosie *Apa.* They have not taken her to her in-laws house, they have only registered the marriage; the father has not had a wedding as yet. She is already pregnant – about one month, fifteen days. She can't eat and she is not feeling well. She wants to get rid of the baby. 'This is a new wedding – it is shameful,' people will say. 'She hasn't come as yet to her in-laws house and they haven't had the official function and already she has a baby in her stomach'. What will people say?

A number of times, health providers shared stories of accompanying unmarried girls, who claimed to be married, for MR services by private service providers. These young women either came alone or were accompanied by older sisters, aunts or female relatives.

Discussions with adolescent women also found that most of them relied on the NGO health workers as their source of support and information when seeking pregnancy terminations; however, there were a few cases in which young women sought assistance from their own network of family members such as sisters, mothers or sister-in-laws to directly access care from private clinics. An adolescent woman shared how she was able to terminate her pregnancy at five months, because she paid a large sum of money to the clinic doctor. She said,

> I was five months pregnant and I got rid of the child. I went with my sister to a private clinic in Mirpur 1. My sister took me and they charged about 2000 Taka (US$28). I paid for the costs from the money earned from working in the garment factory. I lost a lot of blood but I had to get rid of the pregnancy... I was not in a position to keep the child.

MR services at the local NGO clinic

In contrast, the local NGO clinic did not provide termination services beyond the safe period and provided free repeat procedures in the event of an incomplete MR. However, the attitudes of staff and the quality of care remain poor. After an adolescent woman, Seema, had MR services at the local NGO clinic, she suffered from abdominal aches and bleeding for fourteen days. She returned to the clinic to complain. Initially, the NGO health workers dismissed her concerns, but after she persisted, they took her back to the NGO clinic for a second procedure. Although she did not have to pay for the second termination, she had to pay for the costs of the transport and medicines, which cost her close to Taka 50 (US$0.70 cents, the cost of one or two days of food). After the second procedure, her bleeding persisted, so she returned to the clinic anxious for advice, but the health staff blamed her for the complications.[11] This is the interaction that took place between Seema and the health staff in the local NGO clinic in the slum:

> *Seema:* The bleeding is still happening. It has been one month already. I have gone and done wash [MR] twice at the NGO clinic. Even then I am not getting any better. Tell me what you want to do with me. [Seema is brought to see Wasima, a doctor and a senior health staff

member who was visiting the slum clinic, who is quickly informed of Seema's situation].

Wasima: Have you done an ultra-sonogram? Then we will understand if you still have something inside you or not [incomplete procedure].

Seema: What is an ultra-sonogram? I don't understand any of this. I need help for the bleeding...

Halima (the local paramedic, addressing the visiting doctor): Apa, she has had wash [MR] twice and she is still bleeding.

Wasima (scolding Seema): Listen, doing an MR is not good for your health. If a girl does this, then it does a lot of damage to her body.

Seema: Apa, I didn't do it on purpose. I got into a situation where I had to do it; I didn't have a choice. Does anyone do this on purpose?

Wasima (again in a scolding tone): Are you having sex with your husband? If you are, then this can happen and then we can't do much to help you.

Seema remains quiet. She is asked to return on Wednesday morning and once again needs to return to the NGO headquarters for a check-up. As she leaves the clinic, she mutters to herself, 'If I am not going to stay with my husband [have sex] then what else will I do?'

Seema was extremely concerned about the loss of blood and that her body was becoming weaker and would eventually waste away. The clinic did not want to take responsibility for the post-abortion complications and instead Seema was asked to pay for an ultra-sonogram, a procedure she did not understand and which was expensive, costing approximately Taka 400 (approximately US$6.00). Her husband had already spent Taka 350 (US$5.00) for the menstrual regulation. The doctor at the local NGO clinic was reluctant to empathise with Seema's socio-economic circumstances and powerless situation and instead she was made to feel guilty about her decision to have a termination and also made to feel guilty for continuing sexual relations with her husband. Seema's suffering is multiplied: not only did she have to undergo a termination, but the health staff were dismissive of her complaints and instead blamed her for her health problems.

Follow-up care for young women is weak. As one of the NGO providers stated, 'We don't always follow up our patients, it is not possible... some we miss out – but if they come to us then they get follow up but if they don't what can we do?' In another incident, a young woman returned to the clinic to complain about problems she was suffering from after an MR at the local NGO clinic. She visited the clinic twice, but both times the provider who had accompanied her for the MR was not available. The second health provider said, 'Why didn't you come yesterday in the morning? Then *Apa* [provider] was available. She is not here now. You should come then'. The young woman, frustrated at the situation, stated, 'I work all day how can I come in the morning? Now it is my lunch break that is why I have come. I work in a factory ... for the past two days I have been coming to the clinic for my problem and I don't know what to do'. She leaves the clinic. The health worker remarks, 'Rosina [health worker] is very slack; she never does follow up her patients. At the dot of 11:30 AM she is rushing to go home'.

In general, young women tolerated poor services at the local NGO slum clinic and rarely complained. This is because of the absence of alternative and affordable options for their health needs. Observations reveal that the quality of care was inadequate and insensitive to the needs of poor women. Women waited for long periods at the clinic to meet the paramedic, but they rarely misbehaved. Only once did I observe outright anger from one of the slum women. She was a woman in her late twenties and had become furious after waiting for over thirty minutes to see the paramedic. The woman screamed out, 'How long will we have to sit and wait? We have work at home and they just keep us sitting and sitting. All the time it is the same thing: either there are no medicines available or the doctor is away. How long can we wait like this?' The other women were watching her, some smiled and others nudged each other, but most of them didn't join in and preferred to keep quiet. The paramedic had been away the entire week on training and personal leave. When she arrived this particular morning, she was busy sorting out her files in her room. It was 10 AM and most of the women and their children had been waiting for services since 9 AM. One of the health workers was very angry by the woman's outburst and replied, 'Listen you, the government doesn't care about you, has the government given anything in Phulbari slum? It is the NGOs who have come and helped you all! ... Go where you want to go! We can't do anymore...'

This explains the predicament of urban slum dwellers, who are neglected by the state and forced to rely on services from NGOs and the private sector. The lack of options means that many young women suffering from reproductive health problems often tolerate poor quality of services and remain vulnerable to exploitation. The situation is also difficult for the health workers who remain overworked and underpaid and are also exploited by an unregulated private health sector which uses them as referral linkages for MR patients. The exchange between the health worker and the waiting woman exemplifies the existing unequal class and power relations in the slum. Urban slum women and their families rely on whatever reproductive services are given by the informal sector, tolerate poor service and rude behaviour, and are vulnerable to exploitation from many different sources.

Conclusions

Bangladesh already has achieved considerable success in the provision of legal MR services, which are widely available and accessible for poor women in the slum. The study findings from this ethnographic study cannot be generalised to represent the situation in the country as a whole and needs to be interpreted cautiously and in context, but nevertheless, highlights some important issues for policymakers, government and NGOs to improve the quality of MR services.

For young women, pregnancy terminations are shaped by unequal gender and power relations aggravated by urban poverty and structural factors. Young women in slums have little autonomy over their bodies, with little say as to whether they can or should keep or terminate a pregnancy with decisions made by in-laws, husbands and others. Nor do they have any information or access to services, except through providers and family members.

Young women's anxieties and disempowerment are aggravated by the poor quality of care provided by health care services, staffed by workers who are overworked and underpaid. Pregnancy terminations are about survival and making ends meet for health workers rather than about quality of care. To supplement their monthly income, poor field health workers turn to private clinics for menstrual regulation services, which may be run by trained or untrained staff. Private clinics maintain a business, and tend to carry out terminations beyond the safe period and there is inadequate post-operative monitoring. Although providing safer care, the level of counselling and assistance provided by the NGO clinic is inadequate, leaving young women dissatisfied and vulnerable.

All types of providers could benefit from improved technical and gender-sensitivity training, in order to develop a more empathetic and non-judgmental attitude towards their clients and to focus on putting the women and their individual needs as the central point around which services must revolve (Bhandari et al. 2008). Adolescent women in the slum need greater education about MR and the need for timely access to interventions, as well as the risks of performing MR beyond the safe period of eight to ten weeks' gestation and the dangers of accessing unsafe and crude methods of abortion. Health workers also need to be better educated about the procedures for MR, appropriate standards of pain management and post-abortion care and the dangers and problems with accessing services from the private sector. Finally, and most critically, the government needs to monitor and regulate private-sector services, as well as to provide information through media campaigns, regarding 'legal' and 'illegal' services available and the dangers of providing and accessing less than appropriate abortion/MR services for women.

The absence of an urban policy for slum dwellers and neglect by the state create an underclass of marginalised and powerless slum residents, with adolescent women among the most vulnerable. Policymakers and the government need to immediately acknowledge and address the challenging reproductive health issues and suffering faced by poor adolescent women in slums and ensure that basic reproductive rights are met.

Acknowledgements

This study (Project A 15054) was supported financially by the Special Programme of Research, Development and Research Training in Human Reproduction, World Health Organization, Geneva. I would like to thank all the married adolescent girls and their families for their time, kindness and patience. I am grateful to Nipu Sharmeen, research assistant, for her valuable assistance during fieldwork. I am also grateful to Dr. Andrea Whittaker for her encouragement and support both during and after my time at Australian National University.

Notes

1. In reality this is more ambiguous and in all cases observed at the clinic, poor women undertook a urine test to determine if they were pregnant before they decided to terminate the pregnancy.
2. Long-term ethnographic fieldwork was conducted on married adolescent women's lives and their reproductive health experiences in Phulbari slum, Dhaka, between December 2001 and January 2003. Two of

the health workers helped us to access married adolescent girls and acted as key informants, validating information collected. Observations and informal discussions also extensively informed the fieldwork notes and data analysis. In the slums, we tried to select households from the margins as well as the centre of the slum, and those located close to the clinic and further away, to ensure coverage of different sections of the slum. The survey style interviews with 153 young women provided information on basic socio-demographic data, reproductive histories and women's experiences of reproductive health and illness. It was intended to be exploratory and provide a snapshot of the conditions of life in the slum. Fifty married adolescent women were selected from these initial interviews from sections 1, 2 and 4 of the slum and became the focus of ethnographic study. We selected young women from all three sections of the slum. Simultaneously, we also selected eight married adolescent women and their families as long-term case studies, from the initial group of women involved in the in-depth interviews. We followed up these case studies even after the slum eviction in 2002.

3. A small study done on the quality of MR services in an NGO clinic versus a government clinic found an active network of brokers waiting outside the clinics and often advised and took women to various private clinics of unknown quality (Nang Mo Hom, MPH dissertation 2007). Observations and discussion reveal that clinics in Phulbari slum link up with health field workers from all the NGOs operating in the slums and nearby areas.
4. Like the distribution of land and wealth, the population distribution is very uneven in the city. Approximately one third or 3.3 million of Dhaka's population only occupy 1038 acres of land (4 sq km) or less than 1per cent of the total land area, while the rest is owned by the richer families (Afsar, R, 2000). Thus, although the poorest (or low income groups) constitute 70 per cent of the population, they only have access to 20 per cent of the city's residential land (Islam 1996).
5. One US$1 = Taka 67.
6. The struggle of urban slum residents to establish and defend their slums on 'illegal space' is an enduring feature of the city's history. The eviction (often violently) of slum dwellers can be traced back to as early as 1975, to make way for colleges, development projects or to allocate and sell plots to middle-class and richer families and for property developers. Although it is difficult to assess the actual number of slum residents evicted since then, a recent report documents that during 1989–1999, more than forty-five slums were demolished (some twice), leaving millions of families homeless. It is reported that in 1999–2000 over 100,000 poor people were evicted from their slums (ASK 2000).
7. The extent of actual marital breakdown is uncertain because of the social stigma attached. The few studies available suggest that migration from the village to urban slums disrupts the extended family system, causing instability (Jesmin and Salway, 2000).

8. Due to the sensitivity of the issue, the precise number of pregnancy terminations performed both legal and illegal is unknown in Bangladesh. According to the Bangladesh Demographic Health Survey (BDHS), 2 per cent of the sample of 9,640 currently married women said that they had terminated an unwanted pregnancy (1999–2000).
9. In a country-wide national survey between October 1996 to March 1997 in health care facilities of different levels in the country and at the community, overall 28,998 deaths of women of reproductive age were identified (reported). Of the 8,562 deaths associated with pregnancy or postpartum, 1,476 deaths were attributed to abortion. In a national maternal mortality study the ratio of abortion related death and reported morbidities of abortion were 1,415: 30,668 – i.e., 1:22 (Akhter 2000).
10. A Masters thesis report found women rejected by the NGO and government clinics because they were pregnant beyond the safe period. Many of these women then fell prey to brokers who found them private providers who were willing to do the MR service for them (Nang Mo Hom, Independent Study, 20 January 2007).
11. A study in Bangladesh found that out of fifty-three clients, more than half of the women ended up with incomplete procedures and complications and many providers conducted the procedure beyond the 10–12 week period (Hossain et al. 1997).

References

Afsar, R. 2000. *Rural-Urban Migration in Bangladesh. Causes, Consequences and Challenges.* Dhaka: University Press Limited.

Ain O Shalish Kendra. 2000. *Slum Eviction in Dhaka 1999–2000.* Dhaka: ASK Report.

Akhter, H. H. 2000. *Provision of Services by Mid-level Providers and Counselling for the Provision of Manual Vacuum Aspiration (MVA)- (Safe Abortion) – Bangladesh Experience.* Unpublished report. Dhaka: BIRPERHT.

Arifeen S. E. and M. Sangeeta. 1995. *The Urban MCH-FP Initiative (A Partnership for Urban Health and Family Planning in Bangladesh): An Assessment of Programme Needs in Zone 3 of Dhaka City.* Dhaka: ICDDR,B.

Bangladesh Bureau of Statistics. 1997. *Health and Demographic Survey: Population, Health, Social and Household Environment Statistics 1996.* Dhaka: Ministry of Planning.

Bangladesh Demographic and Health Survey. 2000. *Bangladesh Demographic and Health Survey 1999–2000.* National Institute of Population Research and Training (NIPORT), Mitra and Associates, Dhaka & ORC-Macro International, Maryland.

Caldwell, B. K., I. Pieris and Barkat-e-Khuda. 2000. *Is there an urban health crisis? An investigation of the slums of Dhaka, Bangladesh.* Unpublished report. National Centre for Epidemiology and Population Health, Australian National University: Canberra.

Government of Bangladesh (GoB)-UN. 2005. *Millennium Development Goals, Bangladesh Progress Report 2005.* Dhaka: GoB-UN.

Hossain, A., K. Haidary and R. Akhter. 1997. *Septic Abortion: Results from an Anthropological Study.* Dhaka: Bangladesh Association for Prevention of Septic Abortion (BAPSA).

Islam, N., A. Q. Mahbub and N. Nazem. I. 2006. *Slums of Urban Bangladesh. Mapping and Census 2005.* Dhaka: Centre for Urban Studies, MEASURE Evaluation and National Institute of Population Research and Training.

Islam, N., N. Huda, F. B. Narayan and P. B. Rana (eds). 1997. *Addressing the Urban Poverty Agenda in Bangladesh: Critical Issues and the 1995 Survey Findings.* Dhaka: University Press Limited (for the Asian Development Bank).

Islam, N. 1996. *The Urban Poor in Bangladesh.* Dhaka: Centre for Urban Studies.

Jesmin, S. and S. Salway. 2000. 'Policy Arena. Marital Instability Among the Urban Poor of Dhaka: Instability and Uncertainty', *Journal of International Development* 12: 698–705.

Hamid Salim, M. A., M. Uplekar, P. Daru, Maug Aung, E. Declerq and K. Lonnroth. 2006. 'Turning Liabilities into Resources: informal village doctors and tuberculosis control in Bangladesh', *Bulletin of the World Health Organisation* 84: 479-484.

Nahar, Q., S. Amin, R. Sultan, H. Nazrul, M. Islam, T. T. Kane, Barkat-e-Khuda and C. Tunon. 1999. *Strategies to Meet the Health Needs of Adolescents: A Review.* Operations Research Project, Health and Population Extension Division. Dhaka: ICDDR,B.

Nang Mo Hom. 2007. 'A Study of Menstrual Regulation Service Delivery Practices of a Government and non-Government clinic in Dhaka City, Bangladesh.' Independent Study report submitted in partial fulfilment for the degree of Master of Public Health, James P. Grant School of Public Health, BRAC University.

Perry, H. 2000. *Health for All in Bangladesh. Lessons in Primary Health Care for the Twenty-First Century.* Dhaka: University Press Limited.

Standing, H. (2007) 'Gender and Health', *5th European Conference on Tropical Medicine and International Health: Partnership and Innovation in Global Health. Federation of the Societies of Tropical Medicine and International Health, 24–28 May 2007.* Amsterdam.

Warriner, I. K. and I. H. Shah, eds. (2006). *Preventing Unsafe Abortion and its Consequences. Priorities for Action and Research.* New York: Guttmacher Institute.

World Health Organization. 2003. *Safe Abortion. Technical and policy guidance for health systems.* Geneva: World Health Organization.

Chapter Six

Choosing abortion providers in rural Tamil Nadu

Balancing costs and quality of care

Lakshmi Ramachandar and Pertti J. Pelto

Since the introduction of relatively liberal abortion laws in India after 1972, a wide variety of abortion services have become accessible, even in remote areas (Duggal 2003: 47).[1] In urbanised areas, and even in many rural parts of India, there are now large numbers of medically trained abortion providers, although a considerable portion of those practitioners are not officially certified for medical termination of pregnancy (MTP) by government authorities (Duggal and Ramachandran 2004). This chapter examines the complex factors that affect women's and their families' decision-making concerning abortion providers in a rural district in south India. In particular, we focus on the costs, perceptions of the quality of services, comparisons between government and private facilities, and other elements that play a part in the decision-making.

Abortion services, like all other health facilities, vary widely in the different states and regions of India. Quality of care and availability of MTP services, in both governmental and private health facilities, are generally better in the southern and western states, and of course services are fewer and of poorer quality in more remote rural areas compared to urban centres. Health facilities operated by state governments consist of systems of Primary Health Centres (PHCs) in rural areas, plus sub-district and district hospitals, located in the towns and district centres. Private clinics and hospitals are more numerous and generally better equipped and staffed than the public health systems. The private providers account for the great majority (estimated 87 per cent) of abortions performed (Duggal and Ramachandran 2004).

The quality of care in terminations of pregnancy is generally acknowledged to be better in those private facilities that have medically trained doctors, as compared to the PHCs and government hospitals, according to the Abortion Assessment Project and other studies (Duggal and Ramachandran 2004; Ramachandar and Pelto 2004). The wide-ranging Abortion Assessment Project, with studies in six states, found that only a minority of government PHCs and rural hospitals actually provide MTP services, because of a lack of trained personnel and deficiencies in equipment and physical (operating theatre) facilities (Duggal 2004). In addition to the private and government facilities with medically trained doctors, there are unknown numbers of 'informal providers', ranging from traditional herbalists, birth attendants and nurses, to various practitioners of Ayurvedic, Unani, and other indigenous medicine (George 2003).

The quality of care in the MTP services is compromised by the extremely high reliance on dilation and curettage (D&C) as the usual method for terminating pregnancies throughout India. The Abortion Assessment Project reported that D&C was the method of choice in 89 per cent of abortions in the 'formal facilities' (Duggal and Ramachandran 2004). That figure contrasts with other parts of South and Southeast Asia, where, for example in Bangladesh and Vietnam, manual vacuum aspiration (MVA) has come to be widely used (Chowdhury and Moni 2004; Ganatra et al. 2004). It is now widely acknowledged that the D&C technology results in higher rates of post-abortion complications, including uterine perforation, incomplete evacuation, and other serious damage (Winkler et al. 1995).

A major preoccupation of policy makers and researchers in reproductive health concerns the impact of the cost of abortion on women's and their families' ability to choose qualified providers (Duggal 2004; Ellul 2004). One concern is that many rural women and their families might not be able to afford the higher fees charged by the qualified private facilities, and will therefore choose unqualified providers who offer lower rates. This concern is coupled with the question of whether rural people, especially in more distant villages, have knowledge of the qualified services, and whether they will travel the distances needed to access the private clinics (Khan et al. 1999).

In the following sections we examine the range of costs of abortion in different regions, and under different circumstances. That section is then followed by data from our research area in rural Tamil Nadu, in which we present the various criteria and decision-making processes reported by women concerning their choices of providers. Our data show that the rural women of that region have relatively good knowledge about abortion providers, and that the majority choose the more qualified service providers, even though they know that the associated costs are higher.

Costs versus Quality of Abortion Services in India

As Duggal (2003) and others (e.g. Krishnamoorthy et al. 2004) have noted, across India the costs of abortions vary considerably, depending on the type of abortion provider, the weeks of gestation, and other factors. The quality and qualifications of the abortion providers are a major focus in the abortion literature, in India and elsewhere, but it is not at all clear what aspects of 'quality of care' are foremost in the minds of Indian rural women.

A major survey of women's assessments and attitudes concerning the characteristics of abortion providers in the state of Rajasthan (Elull 2004) suggests that costs may not be the foremost factor in women's decision-making. Elull's data (from six districts, 3,682 respondents) showed that 66.6 per cent and 76.3 per cent of women rated provider skills and facility equipment, respectively, as 'very important'. In contrast, only about 32 per cent rated the cost of abortion as 'very important'. Distance to the clinic was even less likely to be rated as 'very important' (17 per cent). However, it should be noted that the majority of Ellul's respondents were from urban areas (60 per cent). The rural women in her sample rated cost and distance to be somewhat more important than did their urban counterparts. The data in that study were from all the women in the survey, whether or not they had experienced induced abortions (Ellul 2004).

Studies across different states in India reveal considerable variation in direct and indirect costs of services. In a study of abortion services in two districts of Rajasthan, Iyengar et al. (2005) found that for abortions up to twelve weeks of gestation, the governmental facilities they surveyed reported average costs ranging from 200 to 456 rupees (US$1.00 = approx. 45 rupees), while private facilities reported average costs from 540 to 724 rupees (approx. US$12.00 to $16.00) for the corresponding abortion services. However, the researchers noted that most facilities charged separately for medicines and any tests required, so the amounts quoted here are incomplete. Also, the costs become substantially higher when gestation is longer than twelve weeks. For abortions in the second trimester, Iyengar et al. found that the charges in the private facilities were approximately double those reported for first trimester abortions (2005: 53).

Duggal notes that the costs for abortion services in Delhi for 2002 varied in relation to weeks of gestation, marital status, and several other factors. 'Private nursing homes and clinics that charged a married woman Rs. 400–600 for a first trimester abortion were charging Rs. 1200 if the woman was unmarried, or even higher if anaesthesia was used' (2004: 132). Summing up the various studies, including the Abortion Assessment Project, Duggal remarked that 'early abortion is available on the average between Rs. 500 and 1000 and late abortion averages between Rs. 2000 and 3000 per case' (2003: 49).

The costs of abortion given in most of the studies are incomplete, as they do not include the indirect costs of travel, food and accommodation for the woman and any accompanying persons, or other indirect expenses. A study by Krishnamoorthy et al. (2004) in Tamil Nadu carried out in 2002–2003 (4,814 ever-married women) assessed all the costs for abortion, including indirect costs. These researchers found the total costs to be considerably higher than the basic fees. They found the median cost of abortion to be Rs. 950, including the provider's fee, medicine, and travel, food and accommodation outside the home for the woman and her companions: 'For D&C alone the average cost is Rs. 1337 (about U.S.$30.00) for service in private institutions, which is almost double as that in public institutions (Rs. 759, or US$17.00)' (Krishnamoorthy et al. 2004: 6).

Krishnamoorthy and colleagues noted that the costs for abortion are further complicated by the fact that many women opted for getting sterilised at the same time as they were getting the MTP. They found that 'when D&C is followed by sterilisation the cost in private institutions escalates to an average of Rs. 3561 [about US$80]' (Krishnamoorthy et al. 2004: 6). Of course the additional costs of the sterilisation cannot be considered part of the costs of abortion; nonetheless, those costs are part of the calculations that the women and their families must take into account when they are deciding which provider they will go to for the pregnancy termination. The combined costs of abortion plus sterilisation are a very important factor to consider, as about half the women in our study included both the operations. A large majority of women who seek terminations of their pregnancies are 'stoppers' – women who wish to have no more children.

Research Site and Data Gathering

This chapter is based on data collected from fieldwork in 2006 in a district in northern Tamil Nadu. It also draws upon intensive ethnographic research previously carried out by the first author, Lakshmi Ramachandar, on women's experiences of abortion in the same district of Northern Tamil Nadu during several months in 2001–2002 (Ramachandar 2003). The area is predominantly rural, and is less economically developed than many other parts of the state. Correspondingly, health and demographic indicators are lower than in many other parts of Tamil Nadu. The infant mortality rate is fifty per one thousand live births, while the rate for Tamil Nadu as a whole is thirty-nine per one thousand (Krishnamoorthy et al. 2004). The female literacy rate (rural) in the district is 45 per cent. Contraceptive prevalence is 45 per cent compared to around 55 per cent for the state as a whole (Dharmapuri District 2001; Dharmapuri District 2002; Gandhigram Institute of Rural Health and Family Welfare 1999).

The research aimed to explore in detail the decision-making *processes* of rural women in their choices of providers for termination of unwanted pregnancy. In particular, we examined the interactions of cost factors with other criteria and situational factors that affect women's choices of abortion providers. We also wanted to understand what kinds of changes are occurring in the decision-making processes relating to abortion, by both women and their families. This last objective is particularly of interest because of the advent of medical abortion (use of mifepristone and misoprostol) and also the promotion of manual vacuum aspiration.

In both periods of research, married women who had had abortions within the previous six months were identified and interviewed with the help of village health nurses (VHNs). Our previous research revealed that VHNs have excellent knowledge of abortion-seeking among village women as well as about abortion providers, as they frequently advise and assist women concerning abortion-seeking. The VHNs are required to keep extensive records of all pregnancies in their service areas, so they generally come to know about abortions among the village women. The cases of recent abortions were recruited from several different primary health centre (PHC) service areas. Some women were from remote villages in mountainous areas of the district; others were from peri-urban locations.

In the course of the earlier study (2001–2002) ratings were obtained from the VHNs concerning the qualifications and levels of 'safe abortions' for thirty-six providers. Using those ratings, we found in the first period of research that approximately three-quarters of the ninety-seven women had gone to qualified and 'safe' providers, although many of those doctors were not officially certified to perform abortions (Ramachandar and Pelto 2004). Many of the ninety-seven women interviewed in 2001–2002 indicated that they were aware of the qualities of available doctors, and the furnishings of the clinics or 'nursing homes' providing abortion services.

During the period of May to December 2006, we collected a sample of seventy-one married women who had recently experienced induced abortion and lived in the same geographic area of the district as those women who had participated in the 2001–02 study. The cases were recruited in the same manner as in the previous research. This time, however, we selected a wider range of PHC areas in different parts of the district. All names of persons and medical facilities discussed in this chapter are pseudonyms.

In-depth interviews were carried out in order to get 'the whole story' of the steps in decision-making and actions regarding termination of pregnancy. A majority of the women appeared to have considerable knowledge of available abortion services, although many women relied on advice from the VHN or from family members as well as neighbours and other women in their villages. Some women reported going to the abortion providers to ask about their practices and fees before deciding. In addition to the case interviews, we also had discussions with a number of key informants, including district health administrators, doctors in the PHCs and private clinics, as well as a number of VHNs.

'Theoretical Data' Versus 'Actual Experience' of Abortion

In research on abortion, as in many other topics, it is important to keep in mind the differences between the 'theoretical' responses of women about hypothetical abortion decisions, as compared with the actual decisions described by women who have recently experienced abortions. There are often large differences between those 'real behaviours' and the theoretical responses of women who might never have even contemplated abortion. Often the actual behaviours, such as choices of abortion providers, are the result of a combination of factors that might not easily be sorted out into distinct categories and clear-cut choices. Just to take one example, questions about 'which kind of provider you would go to or 'what qualities ar[illegible]t important in selecting an abortion provider' do not take into account whether a sterilisation procedure is to be undertaken at the same time.

Because of the many factors affecting decision-making regarding selection of abortion providers, we focused our data gathering on women who have had abortions within the past six months. These women, in most cases, can remember the details of decision-making, the costs incurred, and other factors that affected their choices of providers.

Background Characteristics of the Women

The women in this study are quite similar to those in the 2001–02 study, in terms of background characteristics. The age distribution is about the same, whereas the number of children per family is slightly less, as the mean number of children in the earlier study was 2.53 per family and the current sample has a mean of slightly less than two children per family. Based on the overall rates of decline in family size in Tamil Nadu, we feel that our data are a realistic indication of changes over the past five years. The most striking difference in this current study is the large jump in the women's years of education, as we see in Table 6.1.

TABLE 6.1: Background characteristics of the study participants

Characteristic	*2001–2002 (N = 97)*	*2006 (N = 71)*
Average age	27 years	25.5 years
Education:		
Illiterate	44	14
1 – 8 years	28	24
9 + years	25	33
Mean number of children	2.5	1.8
Per cent engaged in income earning activity	66%	60%
Per cent 'housewife only' (no income earning activity)	34%	40%

Source: Fieldnotes, 2006

The majority of the married women interviewed were in their mid-twenties. The median age was around 25.5 years, compared to twenty-seven years in the earlier study. Our sample of women in 2006 gives evidence of a remarkable change in literacy rates and overall schooling: compared to the 2001–2002 data, in which nearly half (45 per cent) of the women were illiterate, only fourteen of our current sample of seventy-one women (20 per cent) said that they have had no schooling. That difference between the two time periods, we feel, is a realistic indication of the rapid spread of education for girl children in Tamil Nadu in recent years. As will be discussed below, this has also had ramifications for women's knowledge and choices of abortion providers. Although the trend is hard to measure, somewhat fewer women seem to need to seek the VHN's advice about where to go for terminating their pregnancies.

Although not all the women in our 2006 sample had completed their desired family size, the current number (1.8 children), reflects an increasingly strong cultural norm of two children, provided one is a male child. Of the total of 141 children, eighty are girls and sixty-one are boys. The higher number of girls reflects the preference for at least one male child. There is a tendency for families with two girls to 'try for a boy', resulting in several families having three girls and no sons. The two families with five children each have four girls. None of the families have more than two sons. These data are also evidence that very little sex selective abortion takes place in this area. Families without a male child will often try one more pregnancy, but if they fail to get a male child on the third try they are likely to give up and opt for sterilisation to end their child-bearing.

Slightly less than half of the women in the 2006 study earn money through agricultural wage labour and other work outside the household; this is quite similar to the rates seen in the 2001–02 cohort. About twelve women are involved in non-agricultural income earning, including six who keep small shops. Table 6.2 lists the occupations of the husbands, showing that, as in the earlier study, about half of the households are involved in agriculture, although only a small number (twelve) own agricultural land.

Table 6.2: Husbands' occupations

Occupation	*Number of Households*
Agriculture on own land	2
Agriculture on own land, plus wage labour	10
Wage labour on other peoples' lands	25
Various vendors, small shopkeepers, cobblers, bus and truck drivers (3), tailor, and others.	33
Not stated	1
TOTAL	70

Source: Fieldnotes, 2006

The Types of Abortion Services Available in the Area

Almost all rural areas of India have a wide range of abortion services available, although they tend to be clustered in the population centres. Formerly, fully trained physicians were mainly in the metropolitan cities and district headquarters, but more recently increasing numbers of qualified doctors, including many female gynaecologists, have established clinics in the rural sub-district towns as well. Many of the women we interviewed had received their abortion services in the sub-district market centres. Table 6.3 is an inventory of the main types of abortion providers in the general area. This list is quite similar to lists of providers that one finds in many other rural areas of India.

TABLE 6.3: Abortion providers and costs

Type of Abortion Provider	*Cost of Service*
Large and medium-sized private hospitals and clinics in the administrative centre of the district.	1,000 to 1,500 rupees for first trimester abortion
Medium and small hospitals and clinics in sub-district towns	800 to 1,200 rupees for first trimester abortion
Large and medium-sized private clinics and hospitals in neighbouring districts	1,500–2,000 rupees for abortion and sterilisation
Small clinics operated by doctors (general practitioners) in market towns	500 to 750 rupees for first trimester abortion
Unqualified providers with small clinics in small towns and in the district centre.	200 to 500 rupees for first trimester abortion
Government PHCs and hospitals in both rural areas and urban centres.	Costs range from 0 to 3,000 rupees

Source: Fieldnotes, 2006

During the 1990s, the government hospitals and PHCs in Tamil Nadu that were designated to provide MTP and tubectomy services were doing fewer and fewer abortions, for a variety of reasons (Ramachandar and Pelto 2002). In the past two or three years, however, the Tamil Nadu government has moved to upgrade the MTP and sterilisation services in selected PHCs, including a doctor retraining programme. Abortion and sterilisation services are supposed to be without cost in the government facilities; however, particularly in the district hospital some people have reported paying many hundreds of rupees for various 'charges' plus 'tips' to the *ayahs* and attendants in the hospitals and in many PHCs.

The rates quoted in this inventory of abortion providers give approximate ranges of 'usual charges' for an ordinary first-trimester abortion. However, there were many anomalous cases in which the fees were much higher, particularly if a scan indicated congenital defects, such as one case of a defective heart and another seriously malformed foetus. For abortion in cases where the weeks of gestation were beyond the first trimester, charges in the private facilities were sometimes as much as five thousand to six thousand rupees.

Women Talk Freely About Abortion in the 'Era of the Small Family Norm'

The data on family planning, abortion, and related reproductive health in Tamil Nadu and many other parts of south and western India show that the 'small family norm' has become widely accepted, and the most usual way to achieve that ideal involves abortion (Ramachandar and Pelto 2002; Abortion Assessment Project 2004; Krishnamoorthy et al. 2004). For a variety of reasons, abortion is very often seen as a much easier strategy of 'birth control', a 'one day experience', that does not require continued reliance on an unpredictable health care system. In most areas of India today, supplies and regular services for oral contraceptives, IUDs and even condoms, are much less dependable, and include more problems of side effects, than the one visit abortion solution.

So common is the experience of abortion among village women that we found the majority of women quite willing to talk about their own experiences, and even in group discussions, there were often quite frank and open descriptions of individual cases. Of course, that openness of discussion is greatly aided by the fact that abortion is seen as 'completely legal' even though most women do not actually know what the law says about abortion. Our cases all deal with married women: much greater secrecy and sensitivity is found among unmarried women regarding termination of unwanted pregnancies.

Factors Affecting Women's Choices of Abortion Providers

We tallied all the reasons given by the women concerning their choices of abortion providers. Several listed more than one criterion affecting their choices, so Table 6.4 contains a total of more than seventy-one 'reasons'. In understanding the contents of the table, we must keep in mind that for each woman there were undoubtedly several criteria or elements in their decision-making, not all of which were mentioned in the interviews. All except seven of the women in our sample had gone to qualified providers, which is contrary to the widespread generalisations in the Indian abortion literature concerning the supposed predominance of 'unsafe abortions' in rural areas. Thirty-three women reported that they went to qualified private providers in the study area. Fourteen women had gone to a neighbouring district; most of them to a widely utilised private hospital staffed by gynaecologists and other well qualified medical personnel. Those women going to the neighbouring district had all opted for both MTP and sterilisation.

TABLE 6.4: Factors mentioned in explaining choice of providers (n=71)

	Choice of provider		
		Private doctors and clinics	
Factors influencing decisions	*Government Facility*	*Neighbouring district*	*Home district*
Money (lower costs, better value)	10	4	5
VHN was consulted.	1	5	10
Recommended by neighbours, other women, sister or mother	5	6	15
Knew the provider/ it is 'our family doctor'	2	1	21
Facility is close by	2	0	3
Government people are rude, services are poor quality, not clean	0	2	7
Facility is near mother's home	2	0	4
Quality of doctor is good	4	2	6
Provider is a relative	0	0	1
Government rejected her	0	0	2
TOTAL NUMBER OF WOMEN	17	14	40 (7 went to unqualified providers)

Sources: Fieldnotes, 2006. Note: Multiple responses permitted.

Although only twelve women directly mentioned the 'quality of the doctor' as a major criterion in their decision-making, it is clear from their descriptions that qualities of the doctor and the facilities were central factors in the great majority of cases. That is, among those who relied on the advice of the VHN, or the advice of neighbours/relatives, and also those who said 'it is our family doctor' – the central concern was about *quality.* The concerns about quality of services were also evident in the ways that several of the women rejected the government facilities. One 29-year-old woman from a moderately affluent family said of her gynaecologist: 'I know her and the facility is clean and she is a friendly person and we do not worry about the money'. Another woman, twenty-four years old, from a 'middle caste' trading background, told the interviewer that she preferred the gynaecologist in a small sub-district town because she has 'lucky hands' and also she had gone to her for her antenatal care. The Tamil language expression, *kai rasi,* (lucky hands) is the most usual way of expressing the women's assessment about a doctor's quality of care (see also Hoban, this volume). In relation to abortion it generally means that the procedure will not be painful, and there will not be any post-abortion complications. One of the few male abortion providers in the region is especially known for 'lucky hands', and is also thought to be very reasonable concerning his fees: 'I had heard from at least twenty-five women about Dr. S. They said that he is famous and highly experienced. He provides both sterilisation and abortion services. That is why I chose to go to him' (27-year-old illiterate daily labourer).

The women also appeared to consider familiarity with a doctor as contributing directly to the quality of the service. The fact that they had established a relationship with the provider meant that special care would be taken. The importance of personal familiarity applied not only to qualified gynaecologists, but was also mentioned by women who went to unqualified providers.

According to Table 6.4, VHNs appear to direct women to private providers: that impression is somewhat misleading. In several cases, the VHNs actually did urge the women to go to the PHC, but the women refused to follow the advice. Since 2006 the VHNs have experienced strong pressure from the district health officials and the PHC doctors to 'get cases' (direct cases) to the newly upgraded PHC facilities. After many years of neglect, the government clinics are again offering both sterilisation and abortion services. Despite those new developments, including some retraining of medical staff, the community health workers are having a hard time convincing women that the services are truly upgraded, and much better than they had been a few years earlier.

Despite the new pressures from the government health care system, the women who sought the VHN's advice mainly went to private practitioners. In two cases, the VHNs actually accompanied the women to private facilities in neighbouring districts. For that service the VHNs receive a small commission, which hardly compensates for their spending an entire day in accompanying the patient on the bus to the neighbouring district, and then spending several hours at the destination, waiting for the woman to be discharged. In a previous study (Ramachandar and Pelto 2002) we examined the complex role of VHNs in mediating women's contacts with abortion services. Their roles have become even more complex in the past two years. We believe that the low number of women who mentioned consulting their VHNs prior to making a decision about their abortion is an under estimate of their influence on abortion decision-making. This is because most of the village health nurses have been servicing their areas for many years, so the village women have heard their opinions and advice many times; perhaps they didn't feel a need to consult with the VHN at this time.

One major reason why VHNs advise women to go to qualified private practitioners is that they fear the complications and criticisms that occur if the women end up with post-abortion complications. Not only the villagers, but the district health administrators, including the doctors at the PHCs, will severely reprimand the VHN if women in her service area experience serious problems as a result of going to less qualified providers.

Apart from the VHNs, women also said that they consulted their mothers, sisters, sisters-in-law, or other relatives. Others mentioned talking with female neighbours. Women who are employed as agricultural day labourers reported that they discuss abortion matters with their fellow workers during their lunchtime and other breaks during the working day.

Nearly one-third (twenty-one) of the women said that their choice of provider arose primarily because they or another family member had had previous contact with the doctor (and the facility) so they trusted that service. In rural Tamil Nadu, the rate of institutionalised childbirth is approximately 80 per cent (Krishnamoorthy et al. 2004), and other contacts with health services, such as antenatal care, are also quite high. That means that many women, even if they are quite poor, have had contacts with both the governmental and private health services. No wonder, then, that a major category of reasons given for selecting particular providers is that women were already familiar with that health service. In a few cases, women said that previous abortions they had had were also with this same provider. The following quote is typical of this category of reasons for choice of provider: 'She said that she knew the doctor and therefore preferred going to her. She had gone to her for getting a scan. The scan showed a foetal abnormality. Her previous check-ups and consultations have been with this same doctor' (34-year-old vegetable seller, scheduled caste). Another woman said: 'it is good to go through a known source. My older sister knows her very well. The doctor shows more interest and does the job fast if we go with a person who knows the doctor' (nineteen-year-old housewife, married to a truck driver).

Two of the women who spoke of going to a known provider utilised unqualified abortionists. One of them said: 'Pramila [unqualified provider] treated me when I suffered from lower abdominal pain. [Also] I got D&C from her when I did not get pregnant, early in my marriage. I go to her for all minor health problems, and her clinic is just walking distance'.

Six women reported that nearness to the natal family home was a factor in their choosing a particular abortion provider. In such cases, the woman expected to have several days of recuperation at her mother's house, without any household chores or interruptions. That pattern somewhat mimics the practice of going to the natal home during the last weeks of pregnancy, particularly for the first childbirth. On the other hand, the stay at the natal home was generally only a few days in the case of abortion.

Quality of Care at Government Services

Because of the upgrading of some of the government facilities in the area, and renewed pressure on community health workers to direct women to the PHCs for abortions and sterilisation, some of the rural women's negative attitudes toward governmental services appear to have lessened. Our data show increased numbers of women now utilising the PHCs. Of the seventy-one women in our sample, seventeen (24 per cent) had utilised government facilities, compared to just 10 per cent in our earlier study (2001–2002). Although some of the women who selected the government facilities did so because of their marginal economic circumstances, their experiences at the upgraded PHCs were quite positive.

A thirty-year-old scheduled caste woman who works as a daily labourer was very positive about her experience of abortion at an upgraded PHC: 'Dr Mahesh is like a god for the poor people. He made a rule that the staff should never demand money from the patients. He is friendly, helpful and not caste minded. When the facilities are good, why not make use of the services? That is the reason I went there'. Another woman reported a very positive impression at a different recently upgraded PHC:

> *Interviewer:* How did you like the quality and treatment in the hospital (PHC)?
>
> *Informant:* It is clean and the nurses are extremely friendly and they took good care of me. There were eleven cases that day and eight of them had delivered babies ... and three had abortion and sterilisation. The procedure was painless and I did not have any problems after the surgery.

Despite this lessening of antipathy toward the public health system, several women still reported poor quality of public care as factors in their decisions to see private providers. They mentioned the rude behaviour of the nurses and other government personnel, and two women said the facilities are 'dirty'. Two women said they had initially gone to their PHC for their abortion but were refused, as the PHC doctor insisted that they were more than two months pregnant. In our earlier research we found that post-abortion complications were particularly likely in the government facilities (Ramachandar and Pelto, 2004). However, in this research we found only one case of moderate to serious post-abortion complications following an abortion at a PHC (see the case of Vijaya below).[2]

Another aspect of poor quality of care in public-sector facilities is the perception that they give inadequate pain relief. One woman said: 'I did not want to go to the government hospitals because they do not give proper care. They do not give sedatives and injections and they make the procedure painful. I have seen women crying when they were inside the [operating] theatre'. Lakshmi, aged twenty-four, was about sixty days pregnant and both she and her husband agreed that she should go for an abortion and sterilisation procedure, as they already have three children. Both the VHN and her husband suggested that she go to the nearby PHC for the operations, as the cost is very low. But Lakshmi was adamant: 'I am so scared of going to government. Everybody says it is so painful. They are not good; they are not careful'. She discussed her decision with some of the neighbours, who all talked about going to the neighbouring district, to the Surya hospital. Several of her neighbours had gone to that hospital, partly because there is a good highway in that direction, buses are frequent, and in the past, the VHNs had accompanied a number of women to that facility. Finally, her husband relented, and he was able to raise the money needed. She was accompanied by her mother and sister-in-law, and they all stayed overnight at the urban area where the hospital is located. She said the hospital and doctors' fees were a total of Rs.1,450, in addition to which they had about Rs.500 additional expenses for bus fares, lodgings, food and incidentals: 'Call it 2,000 rupees', she said.

Importance of the Cost Factor

As Lakshmi's case indicates, the meanings of the cost factor and its relationship to other considerations in abortion are complex. Cost was clearly of central importance for the women who went to government facilities, as several of them said they could not afford to go to expensive private practitioners. Similarly, the seven women who went to *unqualified* practitioners appeared to be chiefly motivated by the low cost compared to the fees charged by the qualified private practitioners. Women who went to neighbouring district hospitals and clinics also mentioned cost, but in a more complex manner. Several women reported that the services in the neighbouring district cost less than the big doctors in the study area. However, they considered that the amount they had to pay – relatively more than government services and unqualified services – assured them of good quality. Thus, from the way some of the women spoke of costs, it was clear that, up to a point, 'higher costs mean better quality of services'. That attitude among the rural women is evident in the following case:

> Yes, I did consult the VHN and she said that in the private hospitals the rates would be considerably higher. She suggested the government hospital might be cheaper. What to do, to get good services we have to pay money. The nurse had given us a budget break up and why the cost is around 3,000 rupees. We do not get anything free.

Examples of low-cost abortions

Neetha's is an example of a 'low cost abortion' with an unqualified female provider. She said she only paid 500 rupees for the abortion, and an additional 100 rupees for medicines. She chose to visit the unqualified provider because she had previously seen her for a variety of minor and not-so-minor health problems, including a D&C

that was prescribed because she was unable to conceive. A further element in her decision was that the practitioner lives very near her home, so there were no travel costs and no need to spend money for someone to accompany her. Fortunately, she did not have any post-abortion complications. Neetha has one small child, so her mother came to her house to take care of the child. In this, as in most of our cases, relatives gave 'free' help, including childcare, so additional monetary costs were avoided.

Termination of pregnancy at government facilities is generally a low-cost alternative in this area of Tamil Nadu, although there are other parts of India where charges may be almost comparable to private practitioners. The following case illustrates this low cost alternative. Vijaya had originally planned to continue her pregnancy, but when she was about sixty days pregnant she and her husband realised that having another child would put a severe strain on their finances. She consulted her VHN, who suggested that she go the PHC for her pregnancy termination. The process of obtaining enough money for the abortion and sterilisation, and decision-making about providers led to continuation of the pregnancy to ninety days. Vijaya and her husband were aware that the delay meant increased costs, and perhaps increased risks. She said that the total direct and indirect costs at the PHC were about 600 rupees. That included the food and bus fare, as well as money she gave to some of the personnel at the government health facility. The costs also included medications.

The costs that Vijaya listed do not include any estimate of the further costs involved in the post-abortion complications. She had serious bleeding for three days, and continued bleeding for a week. At the time of the interview, she was still not able to get up and do her normal household work and care for her children, eight days after the operation. If we estimate the value of her daily work as 50 rupees, then we can estimate that there has been an additional cost of 400 rupees to the family, which was absorbed by extra work on the part of her husband, mother-in-law, and others. In this case, those extra costs were not a problem because Vijaya's relatives are living as an extended family.

Several women who went to one of the upgraded PHCs told us that they had incurred practically no expenses and had had no problems. Thus, during 2006 there was a significant increase in the availability of low-cost, or cost-free, abortions at a select number of government PHCs. Padma is one example of a woman who chose government services because of costs:

> When I was barely forty days pregnant I went to Dr. Anitha ... She did the urine test and confirmed the pregnancy. She said that through tablets she can abort the foetus. The cost of those tablets was 700 rupees. She told me 'I will give you *mathirai adhuliya kalanjividdum'* (tablets that will produce abortion). I told her if I eat tablets they cause burning sensation in my stomach and it causes ulcer. I refused to take such powerful tablets. She asked me if wanted to have 'real abortion' without tablets. I told her that I would go home and return the following day. I was thinking, if she is charging 700 rupees for tablets, how much [more] would she charge for doing real abortion. I was suspicious about the cost. Therefore I decided that I will go to the government hospital.

This woman was well aware of several alternatives, but was afraid of 'abortion from tablets', medication abortion. She went to a government facility (PHC), where she got the abortion and sterilisation. The total costs, she said, were about 500 rupees for treatment, tips and miscellaneous payments, including her bus fare.

Examples of more costly pregnancy terminations

Kavitha was about ninety days pregnant when she went to get the MTP and also to get sterilised. She and her husband were in complete agreement that they would not have any more children, though at present they have only one child. Her problem was that, according to doctor's reports, her uterus is misshapen, so she cannot have a normal delivery. She did not mention the possibility of having a Caesarean delivery. After consulting two different doctors about her uterus, and paying about 500 rupees for two ultrasound scans, she discussed the various possibilities of where to go for the abortion. She was advised by some of her neighbours that the costs would be less if she went to the large private hospital in a neighbouring district. Despite the travel costs, plus lodgings and other incidental expenses, the abortion and sterilisation cost a total of Rs.1,700, according to her calculations:

> *Interviewer:* You have spent 1,700 rupees to get abortion and sterilisation services. The same services might have been available in a private hospital in the district centre. Why did you not prefer to go to the private doctor there?
>
> *Kavitha:* In our district centre, the rates are two times more than what we pay in [the neighbouring district]. I know about Dr. K, Dr. R. and the Poonam Nursing Home (pseudonyms), but they are more expensive than [in the neighbouring district]. Even Dr. T's nursing home is costly.

The assertion concerning the high fees charged by the gynaecologists at the private hospitals in the district headquarters was confirmed by Chitra, who had her abortion after seven months of pregnancy. Ultrasound scanning showed that the foetus was seriously defective and would not have survived. The decision to have the abortion was made after five months, but it took a further two months for her to raise the money. Chitra runs a small vegetable shop so she is not terribly poor, but it was nonetheless difficult for her to raise the Rs.12,000 (approx. US$ 267) that the gynaecologist charged for the termination of pregnancy plus sterilisation. There were undoubtedly other small expenditures, but those would have been trivial compared to the 12,000 rupees. It appears from her narrative that she did not consider any low-cost unqualified providers; she certainly did not entertain the thought of going to government facilities, although the confirmation of her pregnancy occurred at the PHC. In the two months required for raising the needed money, she borrowed money from a moneylender at 2 per cent interest per month, in addition to which she got a substantial loan from her self-help group (SHG). At the time of the interview, in 2006, she was still paying off the loans, several months after the operation.

A 35-year-old middle-caste woman with three children, who works as a daily labourer with her husband told of the high cost of an abortion which was delayed because she could not raise enough money during her first trimester of pregnancy:

> *Interviewer:* Did you pay two thousand rupees just for the abortion?
>
> *Alemelu:* Yes. The doctor told me the weeks of pregnancy was over three months and therefore the cost was high.
>
> *Interviewer:* How did you mobilise the money?
>
> *Alemelu:* I borrowed and (*kasta pattu molla molla kattardhudhan*) it is a struggle and slowly, slowly we have to pay back with interest.

Malika also went to a government facility, but for her the total charges were Rs. 3000 for approximately the same services for which Padma had paid only Rs. 500. She chose the government facility because she knew the staff nurse in the hospital, so she felt that she would get good treatment. Like most other rural women, she was well aware of the ways in which the doctors and others in the government hospitals abuse their patients. She felt that her relationship to the staff nurse would be a protection, and to insure the relationship she gave the nurse Rs. 500.

> *Interviewer:* Did the doctors treat you well?
>
> *Malika:* Yes, since I had gone through the staff nurse, I escaped the abuses. But I observed the doctors yelling at some illiterate women. One woman was asking when her daughter would deliver the baby. The doctor replied 'why is that so important to you to know when she would deliver? You have admitted your daughter and [now just] forget when she is going to deliver. We are not Gods to give you the exact time'.

Malika felt that the abuse from the doctors was unjust:

> Those rural women were totally illiterate and were anxious to know whether the daughter had gone into labour or not. They had a reason to know because they had to go home and make other arrangements. In the government hospital we are not supposed to ask any questions to the doctors. They are impatient and lose their temper. That is the reason women prefer to go to the private hospitals than the government facilities.

Delays, Debt and Willingness to Pay for Quality

Our data show that almost all the women were aware of low cost abortion services, at least at the government facilities. In many cases they also had knowledge of local unqualified practitioners whose services would be much less than those of the qualified gynaecologists and well-equipped clinics. However, the majority of the women chose to borrow considerable sums of money to fund abortions with providers with a perceived better quality of service, often pledging gold jewellery and incurring high interest rates. The willingness of women to pay for quality is further supported by the considerable numbers of women who travelled to neighbouring districts, thus incurring extra expenses, in order to obtain the termination of their pregnancy and sterilisation. Several of the women who went to a neighbouring district for their terminations and sterilisation were agricultural wage labourers from the low-income category. However, one consequence of this is that several women in our sample, particularly those in the poorest families, told us that raising sufficient money for the doctor's fees caused them to delay getting their abortions, which in some cases resulted in further increase of costs.

Selvi, a 22-year-old woman from a poor scheduled caste family, works as an agricultural labourer. Her husband is also an agricultural labourer. She had complications of a prolapsed uterus, as well as other health problems. Originally, she had gone to a government facility, but they sent her away, saying that they did not have the facilities to handle her complications:

> [They said] we cannot do any abortion here and we suggest that you go to the private hospital and get the abortion services. We returned immediately to the village and consulted 'sister' [VHN]. She suggested that we should go to Shanti hospital in the district centre. [VHN] had suggested that we should carry with us two thousand rupees when we go to the nursing home. That might be the approximate cost. After a week's time we managed to get two thousand rupees and we went to the hospital. Dr. R. saw the previous report and said, *kasu adigama agum* (it costs more money), for abortion it is three thousand rupees, she is weak and we have to give her a bottle of blood and that costs 975 rupees. You should have minimum three thousand five hundred rupees. We returned home because we had with us only two thousand rupees. We had to struggle hard to make up another two thousand rupees. The moneylenders charged four per cent interest [per month]. We had no choice except to borrow at a high interest rate.

TABLE 6.5: Sources of money for paying costs of abortion

Sources	*Number of Women Using This Source*
Paid from personal or family savings	21
Borrowed from money lenders, pledging jewellery / paying interest	24
Borrowed from natal family	4
Borrowed from in-law family	1
Borrowed from friends and neighbours	7
Loan from women's group	5
Borrowed from the house where she works	1
No cost or very little cost at Govt. facility	8

Source: Fieldnotes, 2006.

The data in Table 6.5 show that slightly less than one third (twenty-one) of the women were able to pay the costs of their abortion from their family savings. Evidently, a significant minority of families (or the women themselves) have some money saved, even though many of these women are in the low economic category of the population.

A majority (forty-two) of the women reported borrowing money to meet the costs, of which the largest category (twenty-four) borrowed money from local moneylenders, usually pledging gold ornaments and paying high interest rates. In one typical case, the woman told us: 'I pledged a pair of my gold earrings to get the money. I have to work hard to recover my ornament. I am paying three per cent interest to the money lender'. Another poor woman who had nothing to pledge said, 'I borrowed the money from a private source for interest… I am yet to repay the principal. Every month I am paying only interest'. Other sources that women turned to were friends, neighbours and natal family. Four women received help from their mother or father, who volunteered part of the abortion costs. Seven women borrowed from friends and neighbours. Five women approached local women's organisations, or self-help groups, for monetary help. The women explained that the funds controlled by such organisations are deposited in a bank. Members are allowed to withdraw from the savings only if there is a strong justification. The women wanting to withdraw money have to put in prior notice to the treasurer of the group, and must also obtain approval of the other members. That procedure can be time consuming, and may be a reason for the small numbers who obtained credit or withdrew savings from the women's organisations.

Table 6.5 also shows that eight women said that they did not incur any expense for getting the abortion. These women have gone to the government facilities for free services; nonetheless, they did incur some expenses that included transportation, food, and tips to the duty nurses and other gatekeepers.

Conclusion

The decision-making described by our seventy-one cases shows quite clearly that the women in a low-income, rural area of Tamil Nadu have good access to qualified abortion providers and their choices of providers are based on many different considerations in addition to cost.

The rejection by many women of the available medical termination of pregnancy (MTP) services in government facilities appears to be focused on the supposed rude and unkind behaviours of both doctors and nurses, as well as perceptions of poor quality of care. Several women commented that the procedures in government facilities are painful, because they do not use effective anaesthesia in sufficient quantity. There is some evidence of changes in attitudes, at least at some of the upgraded PHCs. One location in particular is gaining a positive reputation in their area, because of the special qualities of the Medical Officer in Charge. In our earlier study, only 10 per cent of the women went to government services and several reported unpleasant experiences, including post-abortion complications. In these data from 2006, there were very few negative reports about experiences in the government facilities. It appears that, for the poorest women, the option of going to the (usually) lower cost government facilities is becoming a realistic option.

The option of going to unqualified providers was taken up by nearly a quarter of the sample in 2001–2002, whereas in 2006, only seven of the women we interviewed had gone to unqualified providers. Women in one of the PHC areas with high prevalence of unqualified, dangerous abortions appear to have completely shifted to qualified providers. The unqualified practitioners are still there, but they face increased competition from the growing numbers of qualified providers as well as the increased availability of MTP at the government PHCs.

Our data suggest that most of the rural women in this area of Tamil Nadu are willing to pay the higher costs of going to qualified private providers of abortions. Many of the women spoke of delays in going for an abortion as they arranged for the money to pay the doctors' fees and other costs. More than half of the women reported borrowing money in order to pay for their abortions. In the general Tamil Nadu survey reported by Krishnamoorthy and colleagues (2004), only 21 per cent of women reported borrowing money for their abortions. This may reflect some under-reporting, as in our sample the numbers of women reporting borrowing are about 50 per cent. Our data on borrowing may also reflect the relatively more marginal economic conditions in this north-western part of Tamil Nadu.

Despite the fact that many women reported difficulties in arranging the money for their abortions, this did not seem to be a large problem from their point of view, except in a very small number of cases. The women seemed to take a somewhat pragmatic view about borrowing and repaying loans. Such borrowing, at least in small amounts, is a commonplace event in their lives. They spoke of paying back the loans through their continued work over the next weeks and months. Several women reported that they were still paying off the loan.

Our conclusion from this study is that, at least in the rural area of north-western Tamil Nadu, the costs of services from qualified providers are not an overwhelming obstacle to obtaining safe abortions.

Also, the women generally have knowledge about available alternatives for MTP, or else are able to gather that information from relatives, fellow workers, neighbours and others. The women seeking MTPs and sterilisation are willing to travel considerable distances, including travel to a neighbouring district, for those services. The VHNs continue to play a role in the 'abortion information system', though they are increasingly pressured to get clients for their PHCs, particularly the newly upgraded facilities. The continued increase in numbers of trained medical doctors, particularly female gynaecologists, is also a factor adding to the supply side of the MTP equation.

Notes

1. The 1972 liberalisation of abortion laws in India removed earlier strict anti-abortion legislation introduced by the British in the 1860s, following the example of highly restrictive anti-abortion laws in England. The Medical Termination of Pregnancy (MTP) Act of 1971–72 was enacted in part as a response to high rates of maternal morbidity and mortality due to dangerous (illegal) abortions carried out by varieties of unqualified providers under highly unhygienic conditions. The MTP Act allows for terminations up to twenty weeks of pregnancy if there is risk of grave physical harm, presents danger to maternal mental health, and/or results from contraceptive failure. Several other conditions including rape also are included. Although not intended to allow abortion 'on demand', in effect the liberal interpretation of the law allows the termination of pregnancy for practically anyone who wishes to adopt that action. The law, however, is stricter about practitioners, as only medically trained persons (doctors), certified by the government, can carry out abortions (Chhabra and Nuna 1994).
2. The numbers of medium to severe post-abortion complications in our 2006 study are much less than the rates of problems reported by women in our earlier study. In the earlier study (2001–2002) about 30 per cent of the women reported moderate to severe problems after their pregnancy terminations. The numbers of cases in 2006 appear to be less than 10 per cent. We are currently analysing those data to get a clearer understanding about what factors may account for the apparent changes.

References

Abortion Assessment Project: India. Key Findings. 2004. Available from: www.cehat.org/publications Accessed June 2004.

Chhabra, R. and S. C. Nuna. 1994. *Abortion in India: An Overview.* New Delhi

Chowdhury, S. N. M. and D. Moni. 2004. 'A Situation Analysis of the Menstrual Regulation Programme in Bangladesh', *Reproductive Health Matters* 12 (24) Supplement: 95–104.

Dharmapuri District, Family Welfare Programme. General Information Book. 2001.

Dharmapuri District, Family Welfare Programme. General Information Book. 2002.

Duggal, R. 2003. 'Abortion Economics', *Seminar 532* (Special issue on Abortion): 47–56.

———. 2004. 'The Political Economy of Abortion in India: Cost and Expenditure Patterns', *Reproductive Health Matters* 12 (24) Supplement: 130–137.

Duggal, R and V. Ramachandran. 2004. 'The Abortion Assessment Project. India: Key Findings and Recommendations', *Reproductive Health Matters* 12 (24) Supplement: 122–29.

Ellul, B. 2004. 'Induced Abortion in Rajasthan, India: Methodological and Substantive Issues', Ph.D dissertation, Johns Hopkins University, Baltimore.

Ganatra, B. R. 2000. 'Abortion Research in India', in R. Ramasubban and S. J. Jejeebhoy (eds), *Women's Reproductive Health in India.* Jaipur and New Delhi: Rawat Publications, pp. 186–235.

Ganatra, B. R., S. S. Hirve and S. Walawalkar. 2000. 'Induced abortions in a rural community in western Maharashtra: prevalence and patterns'. *Workshop on Reproductive Health in India: New Evidence and Issues. February 28–April 1 2006.* Pune, India.

Ganatra, B. R., M. Mygdeman, P. Bich Thuy, N. Duc Vinh and V. Manh Loi. 2004. 'From Research to Reality: The Challenges of Introducing Medical Abortion into Service Delivery in Vietnam', *Reproductive Health Matters* 12 (24) Supplement: 105–113.

Gandhigram Institute of Rural Health and Family Welfare. 1999. 'Rapid Household Survey: RCH Project. Dharmapuri' Unpublished survey report prepared for the Ministry of Health and Family Welfare. New Delhi.

George, A. 2003. 'From Decoctions to Instruments', *Seminar* 532: 52–56.

Iyengar, S., K. Iyengar and V. Suhalka. 2004. *Situation Analysis of Abortion Services in Rajasthan. Abortion Assessment Project: India. Report from Action Research & Training for Health (ARTH).* Udaipur: Action Research & Training for Health.

Khan, M. E., S. Barge, N. Kumar and S. Almroth. 1999. 'Abortion in India: Current Situation and Future Challenges', in S. Pachuari (ed), *Implementing A Reproductive Health Agenda in India: The Beginning.* Population Council: New Delhi: pp. 507–530.

Krishnamoorthy, S., N. Thenmozhi, J. Sheela and N. Audinarayana. 2004. *Pregnancy Outcome in Tamilnadu: A Survey With Special Reference to Abortion Complications, Cost and Care.* Retrieved May 12 2007 from http://www.cehat.org/aap1/household1.pdf

Ramachandar, L. 2003. 'Decision-making and Women's Empowerment: Abortion in a South Indian community', Unpublished Ph.D. dissertation, University of Melbourne.

Ramachandar, L. and P. J. Pelto. 2002. 'The Role of Village Health Nurses in Mediating Abortions in Rural Tamil Nadu, India', *Reproductive Health Matters* 10 (19): 64–75.

———. 2004. 'Abortion Providers and Safety of Abortion: a Community-based Study in a Rural District of Tamil Nadu, India', *Reproductive Health Matters* 12 (24) Supplement: 138–147.

Winkler, J., E. Oliveras and N. McIntosh. 1995. *Post Abortion Care: A Reference Manual for Improving Quality of Care.* New York: JHPIEGO Corporation.

Chapter Seven

Abortion in Vietnam

History, culture and politics collide in the era of *Doi Moi*

Merrill Wolf, Phan Bich Thuy, Alyson Hyman and Amanda Huber

In recent years, the convergence of diverse cultural, political, demographic and economic forces has brought dramatic, often challenging transformations to many spheres of Vietnamese life. These transformations are clearly evident in both public and private approaches to sexuality and reproduction, as the country's population strives to reconcile deep-seated beliefs and long-standing customs with new aspirations and social conditions.

Such challenges are not uncommon in countries undergoing demographic and related transitions similar to those underway in Vietnam. However, factors unique to Vietnam's culture and history – including rapid economic and social change resulting from its recent emergence from global political isolation and from its aggressive move towards a market economy – throw many such juxtapositions and ensuing dilemmas into especially sharp contrast. One striking example is the role of abortion in both public and private life, which may have implications and offer important lessons for national and local policy-makers, the international community of women's health and rights advocates, researchers and others.

In this chapter, we describe experiences of and views on abortion in Vietnam, focusing on conflicts and opportunities that arise from the convergence of relevant local and global influences. Among other observations, we suggest that an undue global political bias against abortion threatens to undermine progress in reducing fertility and in promoting women's reproductive health and rights in a country where abortion is available, accessible, well accepted, widely used and generally safe. We also encourage donors, international aid organisations and others aiming to promote reproductive health and rights in Vietnam to respect and work within the context of the country's unique historical and cultural perspectives; without this, programmes may falter.

Background

Socio-economics and politics

Vietnam's current estimated population of more than eighty-four million includes members of more than fifty different ethnic groups dispersed across 128,066 square miles (PRB 2006; Vietnam Ministry of Foreign Affairs 2006). For many years, the Vietnamese people suffered the severe, adverse effects of two devastating wars. The first, ending in 1954, achieved independence from colonial France. The second, a civil war with the south backed by the United States, resulted in the establishment of a unified socialist state in 1975, and was followed by a decade of global political and economic isolation. The institution of reform policies known as *doi moi* ('renovation') in the mid-1980s has led to dramatic economic growth in recent decades, vastly improving the standard of living for many, though not all, citizens.

Today, according to the Asian Development Bank, educational, literacy and employment levels are high, with an adult literacy rate of 90.3 per cent and an unemployment rate of between 2 and 5 per cent (ADB 2006a; ADB 2006b). Vietnam reduced poverty by almost two thirds between 1993 and 2004, leaving less than 20 per cent of its population classified as poor that year (ADB 2004). Though the vast majority of Vietnamese live in rural areas and agrarian culture still dominates – between 40 and 60 per cent of Vietnamese workers are employed in agriculture (ADB 2006a; CIA 2007) – urbanisation is fast encroaching. However, sharp differences exist between urban and rural areas in education, income, access to health care and other development indicators, with the large ethnic minority populations in remote rural and mountainous areas enjoying few of the benefits of modernisation and economic growth that have accrued to urbanites. For example, the average per capita monthly income in the urban areas is more than twice that reported in rural areas, and people living in urban provinces are served by two to four times as many hospital beds and three to five times as many medical personnel as those in the country's mountainous provinces (Vietnam Health Statistical Yearbook 2003).

Reflecting the country's history and ethnic diversity, Vietnam's present-day culture blends many traditions and ideologies. Religious practice, for example, encompasses Confucianism, Taoism, Buddhism, animism, ancestor worship and Christianity – all observed within the context of government promotion of the scientific and rational principles central to communism. Although Western ways of thinking and living are gaining influence, especially in the south and among young people, the traditional importance of family over self persists, aligning to some degree with the state's emphasis on societal over individual status. Despite women's near equal participation in education and the workforce, the influence of long-standing tradition and belief remain particularly strong in matters concerning women's roles, preference for male children and other aspects of family life (Sabharwal and Than 2006).

Reproductive health

The Vietnamese government's efforts to reduce population growth began with introduction of a national family planning programme in the 1960s, inspired partly by the need to boost women's participation in the workforce in order to offset men's military service (Knodel et al. 1995). Contraceptive methods were in very short supply during this era, however. Even well into the 1980s, surgical sterilisation and the intrauterine device (IUD) were the only methods readily accessible to most women. Consistent with the ethos that informed family planning initiatives globally in these years, the family planning programme focused on women as targets and on the use of incentives to promote the use of certain methods.

The late 1980s saw the initiation of a stronger family planning programme through institution of the National Committee for Family Planning and Population and assistance from the United Nations Population Fund (UNFPA). In 1988 the government issued its first population strategy and strengthened delivery of subsidised family planning services and methods through a network of health promoters and health facilities extending to the village level throughout much of the country. At that time, it also introduced a policy limiting families to two children, which was enforced by disincentives and punishments such as reduced rice rations and fines.

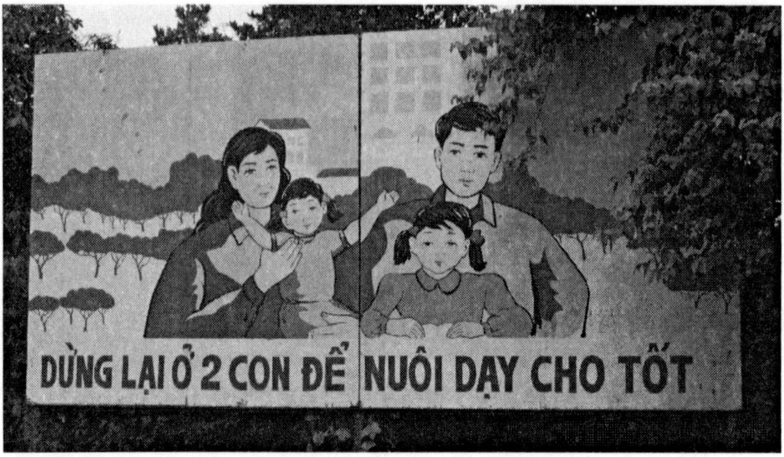

ILLUSTRATION 7.1 The Vietnamese government encourages small families through billboards such as this, which urges, "Stop with two children to bring them up well", March 2009. (Photograph: C. Hord Smith).

Over the years, the two-child norm has been repositioned somewhat as an objective to be encouraged rather than imposed (Knodel et al 1995). This change reflects greater appreciation of the need to protect individuals' rights as well as, possibly, less need for a heavy-handed approach. Having experienced or witnessed the educational, economic and other benefits associated with smaller families, many Vietnamese have apparently internalised the government-promoted two-child norm as a positive good for both families and the state. As will be discussed later in this chapter, some couples do choose to exceed the officially proclaimed ideal family size, often out of a desire for male children or, in agricultural areas, because the benefit of extra hands in the fields outweighs the burden of extra mouths in the kitchen. Nevertheless, the suspicion of coercion lingers around the national population and family planning programme, particularly given Vietnam's high reported abortion rates.

The paradigm shift in health and development that both culminated in, and was driven by, the 1994 International Conference on Population and Development (ICPD) altered the landscape of international aid at about the same time that Vietnam became more receptive to outside financial and technical assistance. Around the world, the emphasis within family planning programmes gradually shifted from numbers of contraceptive acceptors to a more holistic, woman-centred view of reproductive health. The principle of reproductive rights, which is central to this new way of thinking (see Whittaker, this volume), initially had little cultural resonance in some parts of the world where development assistance was focused. But it corresponded to some degree with the egalitarian values at the heart of Vietnam's socialist system and enshrined in its constitution. Since the ICPD, Vietnam's approach to family planning and reproductive health has reflected keener attention on women's rights and needs, for example in steps taken to broaden the mix of contraceptive options, to tailor programmes to special populations such as adolescents, and other measures.

The last few decades have seen a significant and accelerating decrease in Vietnam's total fertility rate (TFR), which expresses the number of children born to an average woman. According to the latest Demographic Health Survey, the TFR fell 'precipitously' from 4.0 children per woman in 1987 to just 2.1 during the most recent period for which data are available (PRB 2006; Vietnam Ministry of Health 2005). As in many countries, fertility is somewhat higher in rural areas and among less educated women; there are also regional variations, with the lowest rates reported in the southeast, which includes Vietnam's commercial centre, Ho Chi Minh City (Committee for Population, Family and Children [Vietnam] and ORC Macro 2003).

Recent data indicate a nearly universal knowledge of contraception among Vietnamese married women of reproductive age and, compared to previous decades, the increasing use of modern methods. Seventy-nine per cent of married women currently use some contraceptive method, according to the most recent Demographic and Health Survey (Committee for Population, Family and Children [Vietnam] and ORC Macro 2003), and 57 per cent use modern methods. While use of contraception increased by about 4 per cent overall between 1997 and 2002, it is worrying that the rate of use of traditional, questionably effective methods seems to be rising more rapidly than use of modern methods.

As previously noted, for many years, the IUD was one of the very few contraceptive options available to women and was heavily promoted by the government (see Gammeltoft 1999). The IUD remains the most commonly used method. However, all but the newest methods are now available in Vietnam, including the pill, male and (to a lesser extent) female condoms, injectable contraceptives, certain implants, sterilisation, spermicides and emergency contraception. In addition, a substantial and growing proportion of women who use contraception (22 per cent in total) rely on withdrawal and periodic abstinence (World Bank, 2006; Committee for

Population, Family and Children [Vietnam] and ORC Macro 2003). A 1999 assessment by the Vietnamese Ministry of Health and the World Health Organization (WHO) attributed this pattern largely to fear of modern methods' side effects and potential negative long-term health impacts (WHO 1999). Some such fears may be founded in or exacerbated by a controversial study in which, between 1989 and 1993, more than 30,000 Vietnamese women were surgically sterilised with quinacrine – a method that many observers, including the WHO, felt had not undergone adequate safety testing. These concerns, as well as others about the study's poor design and other possible ethical lapses, ended the trial, but suspicions and fears have lingered and, perhaps, expanded to encompass other contraceptive methods (Berer 1995; Hieu 1993).

The Ministry of Health/WHO assessment underscored Vietnam's high unmet need for contraceptive information and services, evidenced by high rates of unintended pregnancy and abortion. According to Demographic and Health Survey (DHS) data, about one quarter of all births are unplanned. Respondents to the 2002 DHS survey indicated that about 22 per cent of pregnancies experienced in the preceding three years had been intentionally terminated, 17 per cent using menstrual regulation (i.e., in the first six weeks of pregnancy) and 5 per cent with induced abortion. The same dataset suggests that 64 per cent of abortions occurred among women who were using contraception when they become pregnant. Half of all abortions were to women who had been using traditional contraceptive methods (Committee for Population, Family and Children [Vietnam] and ORC Macro 2003).

In addition to the need for assistance in using traditional contraceptive methods more effectively, the Ministry of Health/WHO assessment noted that Vietnamese women need more accurate information about, and access to, a broader range of modern contraceptive methods. The study also corroborated the longstanding observation that obtaining contraceptive information and services is especially difficult for young and unmarried women, who are increasingly sexually active for longer periods of their lives and who are not included in the measurement of contraceptive prevalence (Ghuman et al. 2006; WHO 1999).

Turning to another reproductive health priority, HIV/AIDS has not reached the epidemic levels in Vietnam that are seen in Africa and in some other Asian countries. To date, HIV incidence remains largely confined among intravenous drug users and sex workers and concentrated in a few provinces and major cities. Its prevalence is climbing, however, prompting more attention from the government and outside donors to address it. In particular, recent social marketing efforts are focusing on de-stigmatising HIV/AIDS, promoting awareness, and increasing the accessibility of condoms (Christensen n.d.; Turnbull 2006).

The role of abortion

Abortion has been legal in Vietnam since 1945 and available on broad grounds since 1960. However, it was not widely practiced until the 1980s. For reasons related to funding, history, culture and other factors, pregnancy termination has played a larger role in official fertility reduction and reproductive health initiatives in Vietnam than in many other countries. Exceptions include the former Soviet bloc countries, China and Sweden – all of which were major early sources of family planning aid in Vietnam. Unlike in many developing countries, during its early years, Vietnam's family planning programme received no assistance from the United States government. When the U.S. Agency for International Development (USAID) did begin supporting reproductive health initiatives in Vietnam in the mid-1990s, those programmes focused on Safe Motherhood and did not include abortion. With the notable exception of UNFPA, the international donors that have more actively supported reproductive health in Vietnam – including the Swedish International Development Agency (SIDA) and the German aid agency GTZ – have more liberal attitudes towards abortion than those expressed by the U.S. government in recent years. The few funders currently supporting safe abortion in Vietnam include the Ford Foundation, the Royal Netherlands Embassy and GTZ.

Although previously subject to the taboos that surround sex and related subjects worldwide, abortion is not currently as politically or socially controversial in Vietnam as in many other countries. Social science studies reveal that Vietnamese views on abortion are affected by the various religious influences noted previously, and especially by belief in reincarnation. Studies document women's tendency to view very early pregnancy terminations as more acceptable than those performed at later stages. During very early pregnancy, many women consider the products of conception as a blood clot or 'bean seed' rather than a fully formed foetus or child (Johansson 1998; Gammeltoft 1999; Gammeltoft 2002; see also Gammeltoft, this volume).

One study found that premarital abortion is an experience rife with stress and conflict among Hanoi youth (Gammeltoft 2002).

When they became pregnant as a result of premarital sex, the young people participating in the study felt compelled to abort the pregnancy if they were unable or unwilling to marry. Many took conscious steps to atone for this act, including by performing elaborate rituals and asking the spirit of their unborn child for forgiveness. Interestingly, study results suggested that the high incidence of premarital abortion in Vietnam is due in part to cultural attitudes towards love and sex that may actually discourage the use of contraception. Respondents indicated their belief that using contraception implied an unacceptable lack of commitment to their partner as well as an acknowledgment that premarital sex was planned. By explaining their sexual activity as a spontaneous, uncontrollable expression of love – even if it occurred regularly – they were able to maintain belief in their own moral virtue and demonstrate it to others. The researchers commented that theses attitudes and beliefs reflected young people's difficult position of being caught in a transition between traditional and modern values and lifestyles (Gammeltoft 2002).

On a practical level, abortion has long been widely available through Vietnam's extensive decentralised health care system. Although the public health system has suffered some disintegration due to loss of funding related to the country's aggressive move towards a market economy (World Bank 2006), it is more organised and well financed than those in many developing countries. Within restrictions related to the duration of pregnancy and the availability of trained medical personnel, pregnancy termination is available even at many commune health centres.

Since the onset of the *doi moi* reforms, there has been substantial growth in unregulated private-sector provision of abortion, often by public-sector employees at their private residences or practices. Other private-sector settings where abortions are available include Vietnamese-owned private hospitals and clinics, and clinics run by international non-governmental organisations (NGOs). Neither the full extent nor impact of this phenomenon has been adequately captured by government statistics to date. Although the quality of many private-sector services is good – some observers note that private-sector services tend to be more client-centred than public facilities – there are concerns that remain unanswered because of lack of government oversight (Nghia and Khe 2001; Population Council n.d.; Reproductive Health Projects 2006).

Vietnam has received significant attention in recent years for its reportedly unparalleled abortion rate. Research in the early 1990s suggested that Vietnamese women, on average, had 2.5 abortions during their lifetimes and that as many as 64 per cent of all pregnancies ended in abortion (Goodkind 1996). In 1995, the number of reported abortions reached more than 1.3 million procedures. For comparison's sake, about as many abortions as occurred in 1996 in the United States, whose population is several times larger than Vietnam's (WHO 1999; Guttmacher Institute 2006).

These findings, combined with concerns about complications and service quality and with pressure from international colleagues, led to government efforts to reduce the rate. Although abortion data are notoriously unreliable, reported numbers of abortions are falling. For example, the most recent DHS data indicate a total abortion rate of 0.6 induced abortions per woman during her reproductive years, with a slightly higher rate among rural women. However, these and other official statistics do not include private sector abortions, and anecdotal evidence suggests that more women are seeking pregnancy termination from private sources.

Vietnamese women's reliance on pregnancy termination may primarily reflect its familiarity, developed over a period of decades when contraceptive methods, especially temporary ones, were largely unavailable or inaccessible. To many Vietnamese women, menstrual regulation (early termination of pregnancy using vacuum aspiration, usually without confirmation of pregnancy) is a convenient and familiar procedure that carries fewer uncertainties and perceived risks than are associated with modern contraception (and perhaps with unwanted pregnancy). Most abortions in Vietnam are performed before six weeks of pregnancy.

The recent increased availability and use of emergency contraception may have begun to influence Vietnamese women's reliance on abortion. Health care providers have even noted with concern that emergency contraception appears to be over-used or used incorrectly by young unmarried women and in some urban areas, highlighting a need for more effective counselling on its proper use. There have also been anecdotal reports of counterfeit emergency contraception products that are entirely ineffective.

Despite Vietnamese women's historically heavy reliance on abortion, however, the quality of abortion services has not matched their accessibility. According to providers' reports, until relatively recently, abortion tended to be provided in almost assembly-line fashion, especially at busy hospitals, sometimes using outdated, even dangerous, clinical techniques. For example, at hospitals with high caseloads, large numbers of women were treated at specially designated times of the day or week, with little or no attention to counselling, pain management or other interpersonal aspects of care (Wolf 2006). As documented in the 1999 Ministry of Health/WHO assessment, other important elements of quality of care, such as infection prevention, pregnancy confirmation, ensuring completion of the abortion procedure, and post-abortion contraception, were also neglected.

Global Dilemmas, Local Solutions

Vietnam's unique history and characteristics intersect with each other and with global approaches to reproductive health, and particularly to abortion, in ways that create several dilemmas at both the national and international levels. These dilemmas merit attention from policy-makers and programme planners interested in promoting women's reproductive health and their ability to exercise their reproductive rights. In the rest of this chapter, we examine several areas in which local and global influences combine in especially difficult or instructive ways in Vietnam, along with strategies adopted to address such challenges, and remaining needs and opportunities.

Changing desires and the difficulty of realising them

One challenge facing the government, international NGOs and others working to reduce fecundity and to increase reproductive rights concerns friction among three important factors: the desire for smaller families, driven by economic imperative, personal ambitions and government policy; inadequate provision of contraceptive information and methods; and a deeply ingrained cultural preference for male children.

As we touch on above, DHS and other data indicate that Vietnamese couples increasingly want fewer children. Although figures vary, in 2002 92 per cent of married reproductive-age women with two living children reported that they did not wish to have any more children; by way of stark contrast, only 4 per cent of women in a similar demographic in Nigeria concurred (PRB 2006). The desire for smaller families is true across all education levels, according to survey results, and is clearly reflected in the steadily falling total fertility rate.

Perhaps even more telling than the decrease in total fertility are data illuminating the Vietnamese people's attitudes towards family size. DHS survey results from 2002 indicate that 74 per cent of ever-married women concur with the government's one- or two-child family norm. Reasons commonly cited for wanting smaller families include the recognition that, with limited resources, families can provide better care, quality of life and increased opportunities for fewer children. There also appears to be widespread support for the government's view that smaller families facilitate national development.

It bears reiterating that Vietnamese couples are making decisions about family size in the context of an official two-child policy. There is plenty of room to debate both the morality and practicality of any government policy that seeks to impose any aspect of childbearing on its citizens. As previously noted, however, evidence suggests that Vietnam's two-child policy is now perceived and experienced more as a reasonable and generally endorsed guideline than as a rule and that the government is focusing more on persuasion than enforcement. A 2003 Population Ordinance affirms Vietnamese couples' and individuals' rights to decide the timing and number of children (VCPFC 2003). Reports suggest that, at least in the past, government workers have been subject to fines for violating the policy, but that enforcement among other groups is not common (Bélanger et al. 2003).

Irrespective of their reasons for wanting to do so, Vietnamese couples' ability to prevent unintended pregnancy in order to limit childbearing is hampered by insufficient contraceptive supplies, distribution channels and accurate information. Although many methods are available free of charge through the public sector and can be purchased through private-sector sources such as pharmacies without a prescription, supplies often leave much to be desired. One reason is that two ministerial-level agencies have responsibility for different aspects of family planning service delivery. The Ministry of Health's Reproductive Health Department manages and supervises family planning services in the public sector, but oversight authority for contraceptive commodities rests with the National Committee for Population and Family Planning (NCPFP). According to reports from providers, poor coordination between these two ministerial level bodies frequently results in a mismatch between supply and demand for contraceptive methods that leaves many women unable to obtain the method of their choice immediately after their abortion procedures. NGOs play an important role in distributing condoms and pills when they are in stock; both methods have achieved broad acceptance thanks to successful social marketing efforts by DKT International and other organisations. In fact, the strong demand for condoms is outpacing their availability, thanks in part to a recently revitalised anti-HIV campaign (Christensen n.d.; Turnbull 2006; Vietnam News Service, 21 December 2006).

Access to contraceptive methods remains especially difficult for unmarried adolescents. Societal disapproval of premarital sex reportedly makes it difficult for them to ask for information about contraceptive methods. Societal disapproval also causes some health care providers to express negative attitudes towards those young people who do request information. Research suggests that young people are reluctant to access public sector services – respected for their technical proficiency – because of concerns about the way they are treated, their privacy and confidentiality. A number of NGOs are currently working with the government to elicit directly from young people themselves recommendations for making services more accessible and attractive to them (Ipas 2003; Vietnam Investment Review 2007).

In addition, although statistics indicate high rates of contraceptive usage among Vietnamese married women, it is clear that many of those using both modern and traditional methods are not doing so effectively and that misinformation and fears, particularly concerning side effects, constitute significant barriers to more widespread and more effective use. For example, a 1995 study found that many family planning promoters and users inaccurately believed that it was necessary to stop taking oral contraceptive pills for one or two cycles each year to maintain proper hormonal balance. Promoters reported advising some women, especially in rural areas, against using pills because they believed that the women would be unable to remember to take them as needed. In fact, only 12 per cent of current pill users among the study respondents reported that they had forgotten to take any pills in the previous two months (Knodel et al. 1995).

Fears related to side effects of contraceptives that are commonly reported by family planning clients in Vietnam include that use of modern methods will make them weak, unable to work, forgetful, stupid or unfeminine, or cause infertility or cancer. Some reasons Vietnamese women report for not using contraception are grounded in local understandings of the body that funding agencies are ill-equipped to understand or address. For example, researchers have documented a not uncommon perception that oral contraceptives make users feel hot – a view consistent with Asian theories on food and nutrition and maintaining the humoral balance (WHO 1999). Studies also suggest that, without proper information about the usually short-term duration of side effects such as heavy bleeding, headaches and dizziness, many women abandon use of the methods within the first few months. Research also indicates that women's concerns about the potential harmful effects of long-term use of contraception may outweigh any concerns about the impact of repeat abortions (Efroymson et al. 2003; WHO 1999).

Another important factor affecting Vietnamese couples' fertility goals and strategies is the persistent cultural preference for male children. Evidently, even many couples who agree that two children are ideal are willing to exceed that family size or take other measures to bolster their chances of having a son (Bélanger 2006; Johansson 1998). The conflict this desire creates, especially for couples who already have a girl, is acquiring new dimensions as reproductive technology makes detection of a foetus's sex easier; it may already be leading to an increase in sex-selection abortions. Recent census data indicate abnormally high male-to-female ratios at birth in several provinces, reportedly as high as 175 boys for every 100 girls in one district outside Hanoi (Deutsche Presse-Agentur 2006; Sabharwal and Than 2006; Vietnam News Service, 14 December 2006).

Awareness of these and other problems and gaps in services has led the Vietnamese government, with the assistance of international donors and NGOs, to develop numerous strategies and programmes to address them. Since the mid-1990s, for example, under the rubric of the Reproductive Health Projects (RHPs), the Ministry of Health has collaborated closely with a coalition of three international NGOs – EngenderHealth, Ipas and Pathfinder International – to improve the quality and range of reproductive health service provision in the public sector. The programme focuses on improving family planning, safe abortion, infection prevention and counselling in eight provinces, with a view towards establishing models and standards of care that can be replicated throughout the country. National expansion of programmatic innovations already tested and proven through the RHPs is currently underway (RHPs 2006).

An especially important recent achievement in addressing reproductive health needs in Vietnam was the development and publication of a comprehensive strategy for the first decade of the new millennium, *National Strategy on Reproductive Health Care for the 2001–2010 Period* (Vietnam Ministry of Health 2001). It outlines guiding principles, objectives and actions for improving various aspects of reproductive health care in Vietnam. Topics emphasised include diversifying the contraceptive method mix, strengthening training for providers and family planning promoters, particularly in counselling, and eliminating incentives meant to promote the use of particular methods. Within the context of overall improvement in service delivery and in information, education and communication, the strategy also stresses strengthening outreach to special populations, including adolescents (Vietnam Ministry of Health 2001). The government is reportedly also in the process of developing a specific strategy to address the frequent shortages and inequitable distribution of contraceptive supplies (Vietnam News Service, 21 December 2006).

Finally, Vietnam is beginning to make an effort to address the potential, if not yet actual, problem of sex-selection abortion, and the preference for male children that underlies it. A Population Ordinance that took effect in May 2003 unequivocally prohibits 'selecting the gender of unborn babies in any form' (VCPFC 2003). In Hanoi, the Department of Health put hospitals and clinics on notice in 2005 that they should not tell prospective parents the gender of their foetus (Vietnam Investment Review 2005). In October 2006, the government officially banned abortions based solely on the sex of the foetus, and in late 2006, UNFPA and Vietnam's Committee for Population, Family and Children convened the first national symposium to call attention to sex-selective abortion as a human rights violation and as a hindrance to economic development and social stability (Vietnam News Service, 14 December 2006).

Strong demand, weak services

Another dilemma that the Vietnamese government is taking steps to address is the disjuncture between women's high demand for services and the inadequate quality of abortion services. Weaknesses in abortion service delivery hinder women's ability to obtain safe, timely care and to avoid repeat unwanted pregnancies and abortion. The 1999 Ministry of Health/WHO assessment and other studies of abortion services in Vietnam have identified a number of shortcomings related to providers' clinical skills, important elements of quality of care, geographic and other limitations in service availability and accessibility, commodity supply and distribution, and monitoring and evaluation.

As Vietnam emerged from global isolation beginning in the mid-1980s, it became apparent that the country's medical system was in need of modernisation, including in the area of abortion. Vietnamese physicians were less familiar and experienced than their international colleagues with the newest and safest techniques and therefore continued in many cases to rely on clinical methods considered outdated and even dangerous in other parts of the world. For instance, health care providers in Vietnam used dilation and curettage (D&C) for abortions after about six weeks of pregnancy long after the World Health Organization (2003) had begun discouraging its use in favour of vacuum aspiration (VA), a technique associated with much lower complication rates.[1] In addition, Vietnamese medical practice created a harmful gap in services for women seeking abortions between twelve and sixteen weeks of pregnancy, many of whom are young, single and not well educated (poor referral practices among health care institutions also contributed to the demand for services after the first trimester). The technique Vietnamese physicians use for second-trimester abortion – called a modified Kovac's procedure – is not appropriate for use in this earlier period and, at any stage of gestation, is widely considered unsafe. It has been found that women arriving at health facilities in the first trimester of pregnancy were being turned away and told to return a month later, exposing them to unnecessary clinical dangers and emotional hardship (Castleman et al. 2006; Gallo and Nguyen 2006; Hyman 2002; WHO 1999).

Other discrepancies between global standards of care and practice in Vietnam, as identified in the 1999 Ministry of Health/WHO assessment, included frequent failure to confirm pregnancy before performing menstrual regulation, resulting in many unnecessary procedures, and poor infection prevention, contributing to high rates of complications. The assessment also drew attention to inadequate pain-control practices and providers' frequent failure to confirm that abortion was complete by visually checking products of conception. One especially important oversight, hardly unique to Vietnam (see Belton, this volume) was post-abortion family planning: women receiving abortion care were rarely counselled about ways to prevent future unintended pregnancies, much less given or told how to obtain contraceptive methods. Improving counselling is particularly challenging given the traditional lack of two-way communication among health care providers and clients and lack of attention to concepts such as privacy and confidentiality (WHO 1999).

Working with international donors and NGOs, the Vietnamese government has made impressive strides in addressing many such problems and gaps in abortion service delivery, in a relatively short period of time. A primary government objective is to reduce the abortion rate, and, as noted previously, public-sector data already indicate some success. But health leaders know that they are powerless to prevent abortion altogether and therefore have appropriately set their sights on improving the availability and quality of abortion services while also expanding access to contraceptive information and services. Accordingly, in 2001 the Ministry of Health's Reproductive Health Department and Ipas – a U.S. based international NGO – launched an initiative known as the Comprehensive Abortion Care (CAC) project to revamp delivery of abortion services. The programme, which focuses on modernising and standardising clinical abortion practice and putting women's needs at the centre of service delivery, has had demonstrable positive impact at all levels of the public health system. Through it, health officials have developed and disseminated clinical guidelines and corresponding educational materials tailored specifically to Vietnam and appropriate for use throughout the health system. Based on these guidelines, programme collaborators have trained numerous health care providers and support staff in updated clinical methods and woman-centred counselling, and in established monitoring processes to ensure ongoing service quality. Other programme achievements include furnishing health care facilities with needed equipment and supplies, and reorganising services' physical environments, client flows and staffing to ensure women's comfort, privacy and convenience (Ganatra 2006).

Key programme partners include Vietnam's two national obstetrics and gynaecology teaching hospitals – the National Obstetrics and Gynaecology Hospital, in Hanoi, and Tu Du Obstetrics and Gynaecology Hospital, in Ho Chi Minh City. Each cares for a large number of women seeking abortion each year; staff at Tu Du Hospital, the country's busiest obstetrics and gynaecology hospital, perform about one hundred abortions every day. Each of these hospitals also supervises reproductive health care in half of the country's sixty-four provinces, including services at provincial, district and commune health care facilities. As a result, practice improvements and innovations at these sites have had a significant trickle-down effect. As of early 2007, the CAC model has been institutionalised at approximately eighteen health care facilities in four provinces, and expansion to five more provinces, with a total of sixteen abortion service delivery sites, is now underway. In addition, since 2001, the Ministry of Health has used government funds to conduct twenty-six CAC training courses for about four hundred health providers from different provinces. However, follow-up at participating sites has been limited because of lack of funds.

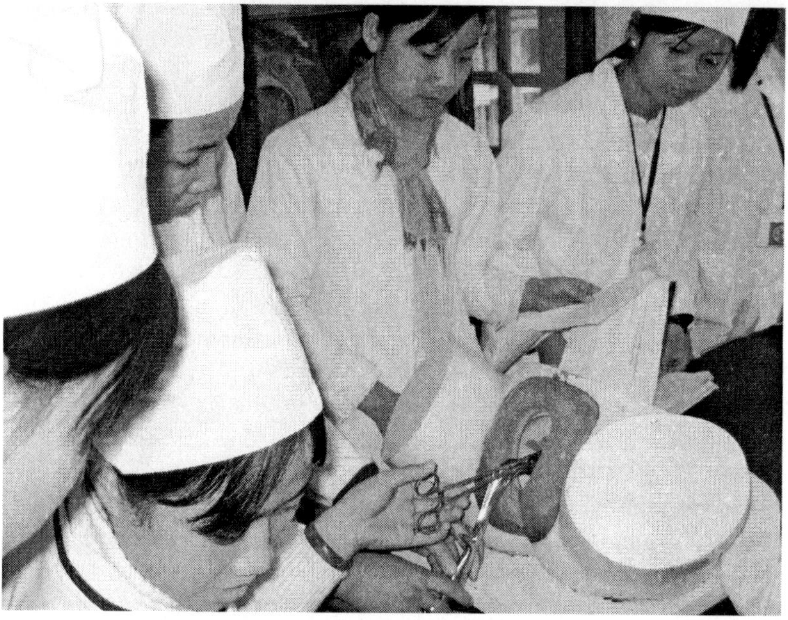

ILLUSTRATION 7.2 Students at Vietnamese Secondary Medical Schools learn safe abortion techniques using pelvic models. (Photograph courtesy of Ipas).

Perhaps Vietnam's most significant achievement in this area has been the inclusion of detailed content on abortion services in the National Standards and Guidelines for Reproductive Health, described above. These evidence-based guidelines establish standards for provision of first- and second-trimester surgical abortion, medication (drug-induced) abortion, pain management, infection prevention, counselling and other elements of abortion care (Vietnam Ministry of Health 2002). A cadre of experienced obstetricians and gynaecologists and senior midwives has been cultivated as master trainers and is gradually providing instruction in the implementation of the guidelines throughout the country.

Another very important accomplishment is the recent introduction of a safe technique for abortion between about twelve and eighteen weeks of pregnancy, to address the gap in services described above that had resulted in unnecessarily pushing many abortion procedures into the late second trimester. Researchers in Vietnam and the United States developed and extensively tested a modified version of the dilation and evacuation (D&E) procedure, which the WHO recommends in later stages of pregnancy and which is widely used in most developed countries. Introduction of this outpatient technique, which incorporates practices and constraints within the Vietnamese health care system, has resulted in improved safety, decreased procedure time and resource savings. No doubt the ability to terminate unwanted pregnancies earlier has also helped many women avoid several very difficult weeks (Castleman et.al. 2006; Gallo et. al. 2006; Hyman 2002)

Though significant needs remain, including refreshing providers' clinical and counselling skills, these and other improvements in the quality of abortion service delivery are especially impressive in light of the limited human and financial resources available for the purpose. The Vietnamese Ministry of Health's Department of Reproductive Health has a broad mandate but only twenty-five staff, of whom only thirteen are permanent. Furthermore, the department has no annual budget and is dependent entirely on ad hoc allocations from the Ministry of Health or other national programmes and international donors, which to date have not been nearly adequate for either equipment supply or training. Low awareness of these needs among provincial authorities exacerbates such problems. External assistance available for abortion pales in comparison to funds for other reproductive health priorities, in part because of the subject's controversial nature and a resulting global political and funding bias against it.

Local Acceptance, Global Repudiation

For all the concern expressed about its high abortion rate, the fact is that pregnancy termination is a well-accepted and comparatively safe method of fertility regulation in Vietnam. The legal status of abortion and the attention and resources devoted over the years to making it available and, especially recently, to improving its quality have meant that Vietnamese women have been largely spared the myriad tragedies related to unsafe abortion to which women and families in so many other countries have been ruthlessly subjected. Globally, unsafe abortion is estimated to account for about 13 per cent of deaths of women related to pregnancy and childbirth. Although estimates in Vietnam vary, its contribution is thought to be negligible.

There has been little financial, technical or moral support, however, for building on what must be considered Vietnam's successful experience with abortion. For example, one of the key contributors to development of the national reproductive health standards and guidelines described above, UNFPA, pushed hard to exclude abortion and refused to participate in related content development. The agency even withheld funds for publication of abortion-related content, an expense that was picked up by Ipas and WHO. In the past, UNFPA has suffered serious financial consequences from charges (proven to be unfounded) that it has supported coercive abortion in China and elsewhere, so its caution is somewhat understandable. But globally as well as in Vietnam, the cumulative effect of such political and financial pressures – many driven by the influence of U.S. policies prohibiting assistance for abortion – can only be to inhibit potentially life-saving improvements to an essential reproductive health service which women will always need.

In this climate, donor assistance for reproductive health has focused on expanding contraceptive availability and use, which is necessary but not sufficient in a country such as Vietnam. In addition, throughout the world, efforts to improve both abortion services and other elements of reproductive health care risk being undermined or thwarted by the current funding emphasis on HIV/AIDS. While stemming the AIDS pandemic is certainly a worthy and urgent cause, addressing it to the exclusion or neglect of other serious reproductive health issues is neither justified nor wise.

This issue takes on unique dimensions in Vietnam, which is to date the only Asian country included in the U.S. president's Emergency Plan for AIDS Relief (PEPFAR), a US$15 billion, five-year global programme to combat HIV/AIDS. Beginning with an initial allocation of more than $17.3 million in 2004, U.S. funding for comprehensive HIV/AIDS prevention, treatment and care in Vietnam has increased every year and is expected to reach an annual level of $59 million in 2007 (PEPFAR n.d.; Vietnam News Service, 24 Jan 2007). Some outside observers and reproductive health veterans in Vietnam worry that this sudden, large influx of money for HIV – difficult to manage effectively even solely within the context of HIV/AIDS programming – has diverted momentum as well as human and other resources for addressing other critical concerns within a comprehensive reproductive health and rights agenda (Le and Nguyen n.d.; Turnbull 2006). This dilemma may have special significance and consequences in Vietnam, given abortion's historic role and women's continued reliance on it.

In addition, there is some concern that ideological mandates and biases associated with PEPFAR funding may actually be impeding the promotion of condoms, a phenomenon with obvious implications for both HIV and pregnancy prevention and which could have residual effects on the acceptability of other contraceptive methods. For instance, PEPFAR policies stipulate that communications (including labelling) related to condoms must emphasise their failure rates, a requirement that one senior NGO staffer working in Vietnam has called 'so contrary to public health that it will sabotage any condom promotion' (Turnbull 2006). Given pre-existing misconceptions and a shortage of accurate information about contraceptive methods in Vietnam, any step that might undermine public confidence in an effective method seems unduly risky and counterproductive, including to efforts to reduce reliance on abortion.

Different Lenses on Human Rights

A final conflict between global and local perspectives that warrants attention concerns a potential failure of understanding related to concepts of human rights. Vietnam has frequently come under attack for alleged human rights violations, particularly with regard to religious persecution and suppression of political dissent. More to the point of this discussion, critics have also charged the government with forcing some women to have abortions in order to comply with the two-child policy.

If true, these charges certainly are cause for concern and action, including sustained pressure from the international community. Sustained investment in expanding the availability of a diverse range of modern contraceptive methods and in improving counselling is likely a more effective way to address such coercion than punishment and condemnation. In the broader context, some western critics may fail to appreciate a fundamental difference of perspective rooted in cultural, historical and philosophical dissimilarities, that may make dialogue and mutual understanding on the issue of human rights difficult.

Western concepts of rights tend to prioritise the individual. For example, internationally accepted principles of reproductive rights and justice are framed in language such as the following, from the ICPD Program of Action:

> [Reproductive] rights rest on the recognition of the basic right of all couples and individuals to decide freely and responsibly the number, spacing and timing of their children and to have the information and means to do so, and the right to attain the highest standard of sexual and reproductive health (United Nations 1994).

But, as in many other non-Western cultures, Vietnamese belief systems and social codes tend to be more pluralistic, valuing family and community over the individual. Accordingly, individuals' personal needs and desires typically are considered less important than family, community and societal well-being. This tendency, obviously, is even stronger in a socialist environment such as Vietnam's, in which the good of the nation or people is emphasised – and generally accepted – as the ultimate goal, even if achieving it requires sacrifices by individual members of society. This point of view comes through clearly in Vietnam's state-sponsored family planning campaigns, whose prominent billboards and posters employ slogans such as, 'For prosperous society, for happy family, each couple should have only one to two children' and 'Wealthy nation, strong people.' In addition, in Vietnam unwed pregnancy sullies the reputation not only of the woman or girl but also of her whole family line.

The concept of human rights may be interpreted through a lens of familial, community and national primacy in Vietnam – as a collective *as well as* individual good. This interpretation seeks a good outcome for individuals as a result of family, community and national well-being. This alternative focus does not mean that individual rights as Westerners understand them – especially women's rights – are disrespected. Rather, they are understood through a different lens. Examination of the status of women in Vietnam confirms this point: although the language of women's rights may not be familiar or commonly used, in Vietnam women have a high status, especially in comparison to their sisters in other Asian countries. Equality between the sexes has certainly not been achieved, but Vietnamese women rank almost as high as men on important and telling indicators such as literacy, education, and workplace and political participation.[2] In addition, gender-based violence, while clearly a problem, appears to be much less prevalent in Vietnam than in other locations (Vu Manh Loi et al. 1999).

In working to promote reproductive health and rights in Vietnam, governments, donors, aid workers and others need to be aware and respectful of differing interpretations of fundamental concepts. Validation of culturally divergent views and experiences of human rights would be optimal; at a bare minimum, sensitivity to them is required. The challenge facing both internal and external actors may be to blend differing approaches and perspectives so that women's individual rights are respected and they are afforded tools and opportunities to exercise their rights in a manner consistent with their cultural context.

Conclusions

The social and economic transformation underway today in Vietnam offers potential for improving the quality of life for the country's citizens, who have suffered much deprivation and hardship in recent decades. A priority for the future is to facilitate optimal population levels for both the state and individual families, while ensuring that men and women can make informed decisions about childbearing and otherwise exercise their full range of reproductive rights.

Vietnam's political and cultural profile, which historically value nation and family over the individual, poses some unique challenges to realising this vision, which may take many years to resolve. For instance, as in many other countries, son preference may be so deeply ingrained in the Vietnamese soul that neither reprimands from the global human rights community nor disincentives imposed by the government's two-child policy will be able to immediately influence families' behaviours in this regard. In other respects, the Vietnamese people already strongly demonstrate that they are willing and eager to embrace new ways of life that accompany modernisation and globalisation and that contribute to families' and the country's socio-economic development; for example, they clearly recognise the benefits of smaller families.

A number of important changes are already underway to help Vietnamese families achieve their changing desires. The government is strongly committed to improving the quality and effectiveness of family planning and other reproductive health programmes, and international donors and NGOs are playing a valuable role in helping the government achieve its goals in these areas. Still greater improvements are needed, particularly to address the needs of Vietnam's increasingly sexually active young people, but progress to date bodes well for future efforts.

Within the broad spectrum of reproductive health related activities needed and planned in Vietnam, however, it is critical that abortion – which has been practiced with more success, in terms of safety to women, in Vietnam than in most other developing countries – not be neglected. The Vietnamese government has dedicated unparalleled attention and resources to improving its abortion services, recognising the important role that this essential health service has played and will continue to play in meeting women's health care needs. Neither other reproductive health priorities such as HIV/AIDS, nor the disfavour in which abortion is held by some influential governments and donors should be allowed to sidetrack this important progress. Overall, efforts to promote reproductive health and rights in Vietnam will be enhanced by greater effort on the part of the international community to understand, respect and operate within the country's unique cultural, historical and health context.

Notes

1. WHO formalised the recommendation that D&C be replaced with VA whenever possible in 2003, in its landmark technical and policy guidelines for safe abortion (WHO 2003).
2. For example, recent data from Vietnam indicate a literacy rate of 94 per cent for men and 87 per cent for women; in India, the gender difference in literacy is much greater, with literacy reported at 73 per cent for men and only 48 per cent for women (UNESCO 2007). Women make up 27 per cent of parliamentarians in Vietnam, compared to only 9 per cent in Thailand (PRB 2005). Long-standing religious and cultural beliefs also revere women. Vietnamese Buddhism's most honoured and powerful figure, for example, is a female *bodhisattva,* Kwan Yin. Women play a very important role in family life, as suggested by the Vietnamese proverb, 'Men build houses, women build cosy homes. And though son preference is still very prevalent, daughters (perhaps partially on account of their contribution to household work) are highly appreciated; another proverb identifies the first daughter as 'better than wealth.'

References

Asian Development Bank (ADB). 2004. *Country Strategy and Program Update Viet Nam 2005–2006.* Hanoi: Asian Development Bank.

———. 2005. *Viet Nam: Gender situation analysis.* Available at: http://www.adb.org/Documents/Reports/Country-Gender-Assessments/cga-vie.pdf.

———. 2006a. *Key indicators 2006: Measuring policy effectiveness in health and education.* Manila:

———. 2006b. *A fact sheet: Viet Nam and ABD.* Retrieved 22 January 2007 from http://www.adb.org/Documents/Fact_Sheets/VIE.asp?p=ctryvie.

Bélanger, D. 2006. 'Indispensable sons: Negotiating reproductive desires in rural Vietnam', *Gender, Place and Culture: A Journal of Feminist Geography* 13 (3): 251–65.

Bélanger, D., Khuat Thi Hai Oanh, Liu Jianye, Le Thanh Thuy and Pham Viet Thanh. 2003. 'Are sex ratios at birth increasing in Vietnam?' *Population* 58 (2): 231–250.

Berer, M. 1995. 'The quinacrine controversy one year on', *Reproductive Health Matters* 3 (6): 99–106.

Castleman, L. D., K. T. Oanh, A. G. Hyman, le T. Thuy and P. D. Blumenthal. 2006. 'Introduction of the dilation and evacuation procedure for second-trimester abortion in Vietnam using manual vacuum aspiration and buccal misoprostol', *Contraception* 74 (3): 272–6.

Center for Reproductive Rights and Asian-Pacific Resource and Research Centre for Women (ARROW). 2005. *Women of the World: East and Southeast Asia.* New York: Centre for Reproductive Rights.

Central Intelligence Agency. 2007. Vietnam. *The World Factbook 2007.* Retrieved 12 November 2008 from https://www.cia.gov/cia/publications/factbook/geos/vm.html

Christensen, A. Undated. *Vietnam's condom revolution.* Global Health Council Field Note. Retrieved 12 November 2008 from http://www.globalhealth.org/reports/text.php3?id=159

Committee for Population, Family and Children (Vietnam) and ORC Macro. 2003. *Vietnam Demographic and Health Survey 2002.* Calverton, Maryland, USA: Committee for Population, Family and Children and ORC Macro.

Deutsche Presse-Agentur. 11 October 2006. 'Vietnam government bans sex-selection abortions'. Retrieved 15 November 2007 from http://rawstory.com/news/2006/Vietnam_government_bans_sex_selecti_10112006.html

Efroymson, D., Tran Thi Minh Khanh and A. Jenkins. 2003. *An assessment of risk factors for women seeking abortions in Thai Nguyen Province, Vietnam.* Hanoi: PATH Canada and Thai Nguyen Health Department.

Gallo, Maria F., Do Thi Hong Nga, Hoang Bich Thuy, Lynn Yee and Nguyen Duy Khe. 2006. *Evaluating the comprehensive abortion care (CAC) project in Vietnam: Successes, challenges, and future directions.* Hanoi: Ipas Vietnam.

Gallo, M. F. and C. N. Nguyen. 2007. '"Real life is different": Qualitative determinants of why women delay abortion until the second trimester in Vietnam', *Social Science & Medicine* 64: 1812–1822.

Gammeltoft, T. 1999. *Women's bodies, women's worries: Health and family planning in a Vietnamese rural community.* Richmond.

———. 2002. 'Seeking trust and transcendence: sexual risk-taking among Vietnamese youth', *Social Science & Medicine* 55: 483–496.

———. 2003. 'The ritualisation of abortion in contemporary Vietnam', *The Australian Journal of Anthropology,* 14 (2): 129–143.

Ganatra, B. 2006. *Evaluation of the Vietnam Comprehensive Abortion Care (CAC) Project.* Powerpoint presentation, 26 July 2006.

Ghuman, S, Vu Manh Loi, Vu Tuan Huy and J. Knodel. 2006. 'Continuity and change in premarital sex in Vietnam', *International Family Planning Perspectives* 32 (4): 166–174.

Goodkind, D. 1996. 'Abortion in Viet Nam: Measurements, Puzzles, and Concerns', *Studies in Family Planning* 25 (6): 342–352.

Guttmacher Institute. 2006. *In brief: Facts on induced abortion in the United States.* Retrieved 12 January 2007 from http://www.guttmacher.org/pubs/fb_induced_abortion.html#3

Hieu, D. T. et al. 1993. '31,781 cases of non-surgical female sterilisation with quinacrine pellets in Vietnam', *The Lancet* 342: 213–17.

Hyman, A. 2002. 'Filling the gap: Introducing innovative second-trimester abortion services in Vietnam', *Ipas Dialogue* 6 (1), n.p.

Ipas. 2003. *Youth-friendly sexual and reproductive health care pilot projects to define services.* Retrieved 12 May 2009 from http://www.ipas.org/Publications/Youth-friendly_sexual_reproductive_health_care_Pilot_projects_to_define_services.aspx

Johansson, A. 1998. *Dreams and dilemmas: women and family planning in rural Vietnam.* Stockholm: Division of International Health Care Research, Karolina Institutet.

Knodel, J. et al. 1995. 'Why is oral contraceptive use in Vietnam so low?' *International Family Planning Perspectives* 21: 11–18.

Le Minh Giang and Nguyen Thi Mai Huong. Not dated. *Sexuality Policy Watch.* Retrieved 12 February 2007 from www.sxpolitics.org.

Nghia, D. T. and N. D. Khe. 2001. 'Vietnam abortion situations country report.' Conference presentation, presented at *Advancing the role of midlevel providers in menstrual regulation and elective abortion care,* Ipas and Karolinska Institutet, Division of International Health, South Africa, December 2–6.

Population Council. Undated. *Privatization of reproductive health services.* Hanoi.

Population Reference Bureau (PRB). 2005. *Women of our world.* Washington, DC.

———. 2006. *2006 World Population Data Sheet.* Washington, DC.

Reproductive Health Projects. 2006. 'Supporting safe abortion services in Viet Nam', *Reproductive Health Projects Bulletin* 2. Hanoi.

Sabharwal, G. and Than Thi Thien Huong. 2006. *Missing girls in Vietnam: Is high tech sexism an emerging reality?* Retrieved January 13 2008 from http://www.eldis.org/static/DOC16286.htm.

Turnbull, W. 2006. 'Uncharted waters: The impact of U.S. policy in Vietnam', *Population Action International Country Case Studies.* Washington, DC.

United Nations. 1994. *Program of action of the International Conference on Population and Development.* Cairo.

UNESCO. 2007. *Education for all global monitoring report 2007.* Paris.

United States President's Emergency Plan for AIDS Relief (PEPFAR). Undated. *Country profile: Vietnam.* Retrieved 12 January 2008 from http://www.pepfar.gov/press/75973.htm

Vietnam Commission for Population, Family and Children (VCPFC). 5 March 2003. *Population Ordinance.* Hanoi.

Vietnam Investment Review. 2007. *Irish senator praises Vietnam.* 11 January.

———. 2005. *Gender selection rampant despite policy.* 31 October.

Vietnam Ministry of Foreign Affairs. 2006. 'Ethnic Groups'. Retrieved 1 June 2009 from http://www.mofa.gov.vn/en/tt_vietnam/nr040810154926/

Vietnam Ministry of Health. 2002. *National strategy on reproductive health care for the 2001–2010 period.* Hanoi.

———. 2002. *National Standards and Guidelines for Reproductive Health Care Services.* Hanoi.

———. 2003. *Health Statistical Yearbook.* Hanoi.

———. 2005. *Health Statistical Yearbook.* Hanoi.

Vietnam Ministry of Health, General Statistics Office, UNICEF, and WHO. 2005. *Survey Assessment of Vietnamese Youth.* Hanoi.

Vietnam News Service. 2006a. *Selective abortions endanger economy* 14 December.

———. 2006b. *Condom demand to outstrip supply* 21 December

Vu Manh Loi et al. 1999. *Gender-based violence: The case of Vietnam.* Hanoi.

The World Bank. 2006. *Vietnam Population and Family Health Project Performance Assessment Report.* Retrieved 1 June 2009 from http://lnweb90.worldbank.org/oed/oeddoclib.nsf/DocUNIDViewForJavaSearch/32555961FEA547748525720D006DE32C/$file/ppar_36555.pdf.

World Health Organization. 1999. *Abortion in Viet Nam: An assessment of policy, programme and research issues.* Geneva.

———. 2003. *Safe abortion: Technical and policy guidance for health systems.* Geneva.

Xinh, T. T., P. T. Binh, V. H. Phuong and A. Goto. 2004. 'Counseling about contraception among repeated aborters in Ho Chi Minh City, Vietnam', *Health Care Women International* 25 (1): 20–39.

Chapter Eight

Abortion and Politics in Indonesia

Terence H. Hull and Ninuk Widyantoro

Abortion presents a confused challenge to the public health and legal systems of Indonesia. While it is variously argued that one to two million abortions take place each year, there are no representative statistics on the characteristics of women seeking pregnancy termination and few sources of data on morbidity and maternal mortality related to abortion. Since the mid 1970s, committed activists around the country have pressed to have the legal status of abortion reformed and the clinical setting of procedures improved, but to little avail. This chapter tells the story of efforts at abortion law reform carried out by NGOs led by the Indonesian Women's Health Foundation (YKP). Since 2001 the group has lobbied the legislature (DPR) and health ministry, stressing the importance of legal change to prevent the thousands of deaths annually associated with septic abortions. They were able to persuade a majority of political parties to support their efforts in 2004, and in the dying days of President Megawati Sukarnoputri's regime, they succeeded in gaining legislative endorsement of the draft amendment to the health law that would have made abortion safer and more easily available. However, it was not signed by the President before the end of her term and thus lapsed. When President Susilo Bambang Yudoyono came to power in 2004 as the first popularly elected President of Indonesia, the amendment went back to the DPR. Unexpectedly in late July 2005, two political parties who had supported the change suddenly announced that they were opposed to abortion, and would now fight the issue as a matter of public morality. The story is not finished, and it appears that the abortion issue will not be resolved soon. In Indonesia, as in many other countries, abortion is not simply a public health problem, but also a touchstone political issue setting up conflicts of identity, morality and social control.

Induced Abortion in Indonesia: Some Historical Background

The practice of abortion in Indonesia stretches back before any recorded history. The earliest artisans and scribes did not regard such routine domestic practices such as abortion as being worthy of note. When it did attract attention, it was related to some important personage, or an attempt to impress a ruler with the description of his realm.

In the cultural context of colonial Netherlands Indies, the guardians of morality were not agreed on the reasons for either opposing or supporting abortion. The Dutch colonial servants were largely Christians and looked to the puritanical traditions of their churches for guidance on what was acceptable behaviour. The native populations professed beliefs in Islam, Buddhism, Hinduism and animism, with all the complexity of interpretation that these brought to the question of pregnancy, personhood and propriety. The one thing that moral leaders of both the colonisers and the colonised had in common was their agreement that termination of pregnancy was wrong because, in the context of the traditional medical practices of the day, it was extremely dangerous. Each year thousands of women died either in childbirth or following attempts to terminate a pregnancy. Leaders thus called for measures to forbid practitioners from carrying out the abortions, calling this a form of medical malpractice. For many of these same leaders abortion was also a crime against the person of a foetus, and was thus akin to murder. These perspectives implied a need for laws to be promulgated and implemented to protect the lives of women and children. In the nineteenth century the responsibility for abortion was thought to be shared between both the practitioner and the woman. Under many laws both were culpable and subject to prosecution and heavy punishment. This stance was codified in the Netherlands in 1881 in the *Wetboek van Strafrecht,* which came into force in 1886. The Netherlands Indies colony followed suit in 1918 with a comprehensive

Criminal Code (called the *Kitab Undang-Undang Hukum Perdana – KUHP*), establishing the criminalisation of abortion. Ironically, while abortion was decriminalised in the Netherlands in 1981, Indonesia continues to follow colonial criminal law over six decades after Independence. However criminal actions against practitioners and clients are rare so the law appears to stand more as a moral statement than a practical tool of social control. Considering that government officials quote the numbers of abortions in terms of millions of cases annually, it is strange to think that the number of arrests and prosecutions amount to no more than a handful each year.

The dusty archives do reveal one case that can be regarded as emblematic of the way the law against abortion has frequently been used as a tool of persecution. It involves Dr Suzanne Houtman, possibly the first Indonesian woman to gain a medical degree (details courtesy of Dr Houtman's daughter, Mrs Madelon Harland, 2007). She was an 'Indo' or mixed race woman whose father was a rich spice trader in Batavia. Dr Houtman gained her medical degree in Amsterdam around 1908 and became involved in the political activities of the Indonesian expatriate community in Europe. She married Sam Ratulangi, who was later to become one of the heroes of the Indonesian struggle for independence. They wrote extensively on issues of progressive thought, but her contribution to these publications is today often forgotten because she used the name 'Dr S. Ratulangi' rather than Houtman, with the result that articles she wrote on women's rights came to be attributed to her husband. Their relationship produced two children and on their return to Indonesia, the couple worked assiduously to contribute to the welfare of their compatriots. Suzanne established a Tuberculosis Hospital in Menado, and Sam taught mathematics in secondary schools and built up businesses. They moved around the country, making contacts, promoting political consciousness and irritating the colonial government.

Officials did not stand idly by: secret dossiers on Sam and Suzanne reveal they were being watched as security risks. Eventually their relationship broke up when Suzanne left Sam after hearing that he had been having an affair with a young Menadonese woman. Suzanne returned to her family home on Java and reverted to using the name Houtman. Whether the rumour of the affair was true or simply the result of cunning action by a Dutch official is not known. However the effect was to lead Suzanne to open a medical practice in a large house with airy pavilions where patients could be healed in comfort and safety. The practice flourished. Before long she married again, this time to Koenraad Schelts van Kloosterhuis, a Dutchman who had been a planter, but who took up a job as a district level official in West Java.

At this point, the records in the archives and the memory of surviving family members become hazy. After the birth of another two children, the relationship broke down, perhaps because Dr Houtman's husband was being transferred to the eastern islands and she wanted to keep up her medical practice. This time she was able to keep her children. She refused to treat Dutch families or any men, concentrating instead on the problems of indigenous women and children. Her daughter still has memories of the bustling atmosphere of the household, of the Sundanese, Javanese and Chinese descent families coming and going, and of the time in 1933 when her mother told the children that she would have to go away for a while and they would be cared for by their aunt. It was at this time that Dr Houtman was arrested and tried for persistently carrying out abortions. She was sentenced to five years in the women's prison in Semarang.

On the face of the evidence, this appeared to be a very unusual case. Why was Dr Houtman arrested when so many other doctors were also carrying out abortions surreptitiously but without similar reactions from the authorities? This is a question deserving careful study of the archives and newspapers of the day, but it is probably fair to speculate on three facts of the case. Firstly, Dr Houtman was a woman, a part indigenous person, and a prominent member of society from a wealthy family. Secondly, in both her marriages and in her young adult life she had demonstrated a rebellious streak, often displayed in direct confrontation with conservative leaders. Thirdly, in 1933 she lacked protectors. She was divorced from a prominent nationalist, divorced from a minor Dutch official, and was running her clinic on her own. To her family, friends and neighbours she must have appeared reckless in her insistence on providing abortions to poor native women. To her accusers she must have been regarded as a threat to the state.

This case reveals an important lesson about the way abortion laws are used in Indonesia. They are seldom enforced in a way that would seek to identify and punish all instances of the 'crime'. Instead they are a tool applied to rare cases where individuals have become bothersome to officials, or where they represent political minorities with little power to avoid legal sanction. Dr Houtman's case is not remembered by current generations of doctors. It is a pity that she has been forgotten since the same dynamic is played out every year or so across the archipelago. Accusations under the criminal code are brought against traditional practitioners of abortion who lose a patient to bleeding or infection. Even in such extreme circumstances, however, the perpetrator is seldom charged. Skilled doctors charged under the code generally are caught in a web of intrigue triggered by jealous colleagues, sometimes being publicly excoriated with charges that they are carrying out the crime in order to enrich themselves. The police, the press and politicians condemn abortion in general moralistic terms, but never face the realities of relative numbers. They are charging one person while at the same time they say there are millions of abortions being carried out. It is in this context that feminist organisations have for decades called for reform of the legal provisions that are used to harass doctors but fail to protect women. To understand their arguments, we need to consider how laws and policies have been made in the six decades of Indonesian independence.

Structures of Governance and Politics of Governing Independent Indonesia

The Indonesian Constitution of 1945 provided the foundation for the formation and workings of the government of the Republic, but this foundation was often shaken and sometimes ignored. The original design was relatively straightforward, and was based on institutional forms familiar to European governments. There were three branches of state: the legislature in the form of the People's Representative Assembly (*Dewan Perwakilan Rakyat* or DPR) to make laws; the executive under the control of the President to carry out laws; and the judiciary in the form of the highest court, the *Mahkamah Agung* (MA) to interpret and apply laws. The branches hold equal status though they obviously have different powers in line with the functions they perform. Indonesia instituted the People's Consultative Assembly (*Majelis Perwakilan Rakyat* or MPR) to oversee this structure. It consists of the members of the DPR and additional members drawn from various social organisations or functional groups. The MPR was responsible for the selection of the President and the confirmation of the membership of the MA. It is the MPR that is responsible for any amendments to the Constitution.

While each branch was given distinctive powers with the intention that there would be checks and balances in the exercise of power, from the earliest days there were frequently conflicts as leaders jockeyed for advantage in struggles between different political groupings across the nation. A proliferation of political parties based on religion, ethnicity or culture exacerbated tensions as participants appealed to identity rather than ideology to define their interests.

Sukarno, the first President of the Republic, regarded the structure and value base of the 1945 Constitution as too Western and unwieldy. He pressed for various amendments throughout the 1950s but political parties were jealous of the control they could muster in the DPR and resisted the blandishments of the President. Coalitions of interests waxed and waned and Indonesia found itself buffeted by influences of the Cold War with foreign powers vying to write their own interests in Indonesian institutions. The U.S.A. and European countries supported the military and some liberal political parties while the USSR and the People's Republic of China poured resources into the Indonesian Communist Party (*Partai Komunis Indonesia* — PKI) and supported many initiatives of President Sukarno. In the course of this rambunctious action the President moved to neuter the DPR and control the MA to concentrate power in the hands of the executive. He also attempted to project Indonesia into a position of world leadership with collaborations across Asia and Africa. Issues of health, education and economic development at home took a back-seat to global politics. While there were many professionals and community groups calling for action to address maternal mortality through the provision of contraception, the government ignored the daily routine of women's distressing reproductive health, taking notice only when a case threatened to have a political impact.

Tensions building through the 1950s and early 1960s exploded in 1965 with an ill-defined attempted coup that precipitated a sea change in Indonesian politics. Over the course of two years, the PKI was outlawed and millions of its members and supporters either killed or imprisoned. Sukarno hung on to the title of President for a while, but his powers were usurped by a group of military leaders. In 1966 General Suharto assumed most of the powers of the presidency and formed a New Order government with a hastily convened 'provisional' MPR. In March 1967, he was appointed the 'Acting President' and in 1968 was elected to the first of six five-year terms that he was to serve before being toppled in May 1998, just months into his seventh elected term. Where Sukarno had pushed aside the DPR, Suharto and his supporters saw advantage in giving formal acknowledgement to the institution, while ensuring that the members remained totally loyal and unquestioning of the executive.

Political parties were rolled into two aggregate groupings roughly representing nationalist and Islamic interests. A huge organisation of 'Functional Groups' called GOLKAR was formed; mass membership included all civil servants and military and it became the political vehicle to contest elections. Suharto treated the entire bureaucracy and legislature like a military unit and instituted a web of training activities to foster discipline, uniformity and commitment to the basic principles of a secular political system. The New Order saw the emergence of very strong, centralised systems of governance, and these fostered improvements in health, education and economic prosperity. Nonetheless, some underlying ethnic, religious and personal tensions remained close to the surface, producing regular blemishes on the idea of political stability. It was in this context that reproductive health policy was shaped.

The Abortion Debate in the Political Maelstrom

Over the course of both the Old and New Order, abortion was a constant irritant to the body politic. While never dominating the political debates of the time, it was an abiding problem. In the 1950s contraceptive technologies were crude, only a handful of doctors were trained to assist women with fertility control, and politicians like Sukarno were quoted in public as being supporters of high fertility as a means of expanding the national workforce. In the 1970s, the development of the oral contraceptive pill made birth control cheaper and more effective. The establishment of international assistance agencies to promote family planning guided countries like Indonesia into programmes of population control. Abortion was problematic in this time of transition. In Jakarta, groups of doctors campaigned to prevent septic abortion deaths through the legalisation of medically indicated procedures. In 1964, the Indonesian Association of Obstetrics and Gynaecology and the Indonesian Medical Association held a symposium to discuss the impact that illegal abortions had on the rate of maternal mortality. A decade later the *Indonesian Journal of Obstetrics and Gynaecology* published a special issue (vol. 1 no. 2) on abortion, in honour of the 1974 United Nations Population Year. The presentations in both venues were consistent in a number of ways. There was recognition that unsafe abortions were a major cause of maternal morbidity and mortality. Hospital maternity wards were found to be straining from the pressure of septic abortions. Doctors were limited by law in what they could do to prevent these problems but they were also concerned about the implications if they did not provide safe pregnancy termination. In the absence of full legalisation, they sought protection from the courts to avoid prosecution for what was regarded as a vital medical need in Indonesia.

The United States Agency for International Development (USAID) provided assistance around some of these dilemmas. Equipment to support vacuum aspiration, or what came to be called menstrual regulation (MR), was distributed across the country. Paramedics and doctors were trained to carry out safe procedures on women between six and fourteen weeks' gestation. A technical distinction was made between the concept of inducing a delayed menstruation (MR) and termination of an established pregnancy (abortion). For doctors carrying out the procedures, however, it was clear that a conception had occurred and in most cases pregnancy was well established. However, in the absence of a positive pregnancy test the patient and the doctor could maintain the assumption that a delayed period was being regulated, rather than a pregnancy terminated.

Students in medical schools were taught the new techniques, and over the course of the 1970s it became easier for urban residents to find a doctor who would provide a safe abortion, even if the name had been changed to MR. For a time it appeared that the stipulations of the criminal code would be overcome by a combination of new technology and assiduous coalition building. Doctors and lawyers pressed the Attorney General, Justices of the High Court and government Ministers to accept MR as a medically approved procedure, while continuing the criminal sanctions against abortions carried out by non-medically trained people. Word spread among the medical profession that prosecutions would not occur so long as procedures adhered to high medical standards and no harm was done to the woman.

This informal compromise might well have progressed to firm case law in Indonesia but for two developments: the rise of conservative policies in the United States, which resulted in the reversal of programmes of development assistance for MR, and a related rise in active policies opposing abortion. While American Right to Life debates were not widely known or understood in the Indonesian community, the impact of anti-abortion rhetoric was strongly reflected in the international conferences and meetings attended by Indonesian policy-makers.

First Attempts at Legal Reform

The medical professions in Indonesia found the inconsistencies in policy carried out by the national family planning programme to be both vexatious and potentially dangerous to doctors. Protection for abortion activities was initially offered by the government policy of birth control so long as the USAID programme of training was in place. However, it evaporated when the international debate changed direction with the so-called Mexico City Policy under President Ronald Reagan. During the 1980s international attacks on abortion rights reshaped the critical environment for domestic debates in countries that shared none of the political context supporting the American positions. Many political forces took up anti-abortion positions as a means of establishing identities defined by opposition to any governmental efforts to use liberalised abortion laws to promote women's welfare.

In Indonesia, it was Islamic groups that took such positions to oppose the New Order government. The family planning programme was charged with contributing to lax morality by promoting 'free sex and abortion'. While Suharto had a firm grip on power, such critiques were muted and could not substantially inhibit the contraception programme, but they did draw attention to the abortion provisions in the criminal code. For many citizens the discussion served to sharpen the questions about the rule of law and the roles of religion in a country enjoying unprecedented economic growth.

Advocates for family planning and safe abortion faced a dilemma. On the one hand they were not enamoured of the authoritarian government and agreed with many of the criticisms put by Islamic groups. On the other hand, even though they shared many of the religious beliefs and moral values of the critics, they placed much greater stress on the plight of women. Consequently they embarked on a complicated strategy to coopt the largest Islamic groups to support the cause of women's reproductive health, while at the same time lobbying government departments to change the legal framework surrounding the issue of abortion. Throughout the 1990s they pursued an active programme of workshops, publications and public discussions to promote their aims, often with funding from international NGOs, UN agencies and sympathetic government units.

In both these strategies they initially experienced moderate success. Activists from the largest Muslim mass organisations, *Nahdlatul Ulama* (NU) and *Muhammadiyah*, were enlisted into the cause of improved reproductive health care for women, including support for safe abortion. While they did not reflect the ideology of more fundamentalist groups, the fact that they were able to bring the imprimatur of orthodox Islam to the advocacy meant that the debate surrounding the implementation of the 1994 ICPD Programme of Action could not simply be dismissed as a 'Western' plot. Reproductive health had been re-defined as a central issue for socially minded Muslims. With this broader constituency, the call for legal change to deal with unsafe abortion became less of a touchstone issue of political conflict. The first opportunity for reform came as the DPR considered a draft law concerning health. While this could best be described as an aspirational statute rather than black-letter law, it opened an opportunity for abortion to be shifted from a criminal issue to one of medical regulation. Working with the Department of Health, activists pressed for a statement that would make abortion legal if performed by licensed, trained medical personnel. The DPR in 1991–2 was no longer the supine institution that Suharto had maintained since 1971. Review of laws in the committee system was increasingly fractious. When the Draft Health Law was examined by legislators, they immediately challenged both the language and the content of the clauses touching on abortion. Transcripts showed arguments from Islamic and military factions questioning the propriety of any steps that would legalise abortion.

Officials from the Department of Health and advocates of reproductive health were shocked to see the law that emerged from the DPR (see Appendix 8.1). The so-called rubber stamp turned out to be a sledgehammer. The word *'aborsi'* in the Department of Health's draft had disappeared completely and instead of liberalising the situation, the final draft appeared to reconfirm that abortion was criminal, and the neologism 'certain medical procedures' would be a practice that was severely regulated. What these procedures might be was unclear, since they were said to be related to saving the life of a mother and/or her foetus, a nonsensical perspective when talking about pregnancy termination. With the Health Law of 1992 abortion had become illegal through two statutes – the colonial criminal code and the confusing health law.

The impact on women was not as great as might have been expected. Indonesians had grown used to laws that appeared strict but could be 'managed' in everyday life. The legal confusion offered more loopholes for doctors, more opportunities for graft by police officers, and more cynicism among the activists. When we published a paper highlighting the problems of the 1992 Health Law (Hull,

Widyantoro, and Sarsanto 1993) colleagues in Indonesia were bemused. They could see that the system was dysfunctional, but they argued that so long as Indonesia was ruled by ignorant legislators and an authoritarian president, dysfunction offered protection to progressives.

Transition to Hope

The collapse of the New Order government in 1998 inflated the hopes of intellectuals and activists. Suharto's reputation appeared to have gone from 'Smiling General' to 'ex-dictator' overnight, and throughout Jakarta reformers looked to a future of democratic development. Among those with sharpened ambitions were feminists and public health professionals. Although the new government contained many old faces from the New Order, there was no denying that the spirit of the time was characterised by talk of reform. Abortion was not the central concern of politicians, but it remained on the back burner, bubbling away with regular meetings discussing the tragedy of maternal mortality caused by the all-too-common occurrence of unsafe abortion. The discussions took on a new character, however, with increasing attention to numbers, as demographers and epidemiologists pointed out the population dimension of pregnancy termination with calculations aimed at clarifying the human dimensions of the problem.

Estimates of Abortion at the Turn of the Century

While discussions of abortion had been regularly held between the 1960s and the 1980s, it was only in the 1990s that serious attempts were made to estimate the annual number of terminations. In part this was the result of a shift away from the clinical to the population perspective. While doctors could easily describe the phenomenon in terms of septic abortion patients in hospital or characteristics of women coming through the semi-legal clinical services, the concept of abortion rates and ratios was beyond their grasp.

Our attempt to estimate the annual number of procedures in 1993 (Table 8.1) arose out of frustration felt in observing the debates over the 1992 Health Law. Parliamentarians seemed to have no understanding of the immensity of the issue. Our estimate of 750,000 procedures appeared large in comparison with the estimated five

TABLE 8.1 Estimates of annual numbers of abortions in Indonesia

Time	*Estimate of Annual Incidence of Induced Abortion*	*Method of estimation*	*Source*
1992	750,000 to 1 million	Inference from numbers of professionals and traditional providers multiplied by assumed numbers of cases per provider.	Hull, Widyantoro and Sarsanto 1993.
1999	1.3 million induced and 1 million spontaneous	Survey of four sites (n=529)	Association of Obstetricians and Gynaecologists (POGI) and Department of Health (Jakarta Post 2000)
2000	2 million (induced and spontaneous)	Service Delivery point social mapping	UNFPA funded study (Utomo et al. 2002)
2002	2.5 to 3.0 million	Using a 'tip of the iceberg' reasoning: If the measured number was 2 million, then the real number must be bigger.	Tjitarsa (*Kompas* 2002)
2005	2.3 million	No method indicated.	Azrul Azwar (Mitra Inti Indonesia 2005: 97)

million births each year. While our estimate was impossible to substantiate, it had the benefit of being based on logical assumptions about the sort of practitioners who were known to carry out abortions, and reasonable assumptions about the proportion that did so regularly. At the time we argued that any alternatives to these estimates would have to be based on detailed research at the community level.

Within months newspapers were quoting experts who took our estimate as a base and inflated the numbers upwards, on the theory that any estimate would have been conservative and the numbers would naturally rise rapidly. Certainly the estimates were changing the nature of the debate. It was possible to use the estimates of total procedures to say something about the relative importance of different types of providers and the characteristics of the women demanding the services. Whether the estimate was 750,000 or 1.2 million, it was clear that most abortions were provided to married women, not the stereotypical unmarried teenager. Also, it was likely that large numbers of procedures were conducted by people who had no medical training, sometimes in ways designed to simply provoke bleeding so women could go to hospital to have the abortion completed by a trained professional. With those parameters set, the case studies published by clinicians concerning septic abortions had a firmer context than had been possible previously.

The most reliable estimate of abortion numbers was carried out in 2000 and 2001 by Budi Utomo and colleagues working across the country in urban and rural settings. Using an innovative approach to verify the reports of selected service providers, they calculated that a minimum of two million abortions occurred in 2000 of which over half were induced and around 40 per cent were spontaneous. Just as in 1993 it didn't take long before experts, including staff of the Department of Health, were misquoting the data to imply that there were two million induced abortions annually.

Fired up by the figures appearing in Table 8.1, activists campaigning for legal change became increasingly hopeful that lawmakers would reconsider the situation of abortion in the criminal code and the confusions of the 1992 Health Law. They believed that the Reform Era beginning in 1998 would live up to its name and women would gain the protection of certainty under law and access to safe abortion technologies.

Catalysts for Abortion Law Reform

The removal of the leader who had maintained authoritarian constraints did not mean that democratic rights would arise automatically. The basic institutions of government established in the 1945 Constitution of Independent Indonesia needed to be reinvented, and in this context all attempts at reform required changes in procedures and the webs of relationships in government. In the New Order period of President Suharto, the DPR had grown increasingly restive and many members had ambitions of power based on more than patronage. Parties chafed under the goading of presidential instructions and mass membership threw up candidates for election who increasingly regarded the votes they received as a mandate to represent their followers rather than their leaders.

The transition from New Order to Reform Era took place in 1998 during a period of street riots, mass protest and anger over the collapse of the economy. Suharto's allies deserted him, and on May 20 he announced to the nation that he was stepping down. The following day Vice President Habibie took control, and soon after confirmed a Cabinet consisting largely of previous Suharto appointees. In the subsequent three presidents' terms (Habibie, Wahid and Sukarnoputri) the DPR became the main stage for the reconstruction of democratic institutions while the executive branch remained a haven for New Order–era officials. At the same time, the call for reform encouraged members of the executive branch to embark in directions very different from Suharto's. While there may not have been much change in the players, they proposed changes that were startlingly dramatic.

In January 1999, President Habibie announced a referendum in East Timor to decide on the fate of the province. He appeared to be simply fed up over the international criticism of Indonesian rule in the territory, and assumed that the Timorese would confirm his belief that Indonesia was popular in Dili. They did not. Tragically, this led to violence which marred the creation of an independent Timor Leste in 2002 and tarnished Indonesia's international reputation. It also discredited ABRI (the armed forces), eventually leading to a transformation of the military into the TNI (Indonesian National Military) the separation of the police force into an autonomous unit, and the de-politicisation of the forces.

In February 1999, the DPR passed a law allowing the free establishment of political parties. Within weeks over forty parties were formed to contest legislative elections scheduled for later in the year. In May 1999 laws creating a radically decentralised governmental system were passed, with provisions to shift most government functions from the central government to the level of the district, thus bypassing the province. At face value, these laws overthrew Suharto's carefully crafted authoritarianism.

By October 1999, such changes had begun to show results in the transformation of the government. A new MPR and DPR had been elected by popular vote for candidates from the newly formed parties. The MPR selected Abdurrahman Wahid as President with Megawati Sukarnoputri as Vice President. There was hope that democracy would pave the way to social reform. Among those pushing for change were the feminist activists inspired by the 1994 Cairo Conference on Population and Development. They called for a human rights–based reproductive health policy in contrast to the population control principles underlying the New Order family planning programme. They hoped that the Wahid regime and a rejuvenated DPR would embrace these ideas, and they were delighted when the President appointed a young, energetic woman to be responsible for women's issues as the Minister for Women's Empowerment. This was particularly interesting when it was revealed that she had set a condition that she would take the post only if it included responsibility for the National Family Planning Program, and that she had the intention to use this position to promote reproductive rights. The activists were somewhat cautious, however, because the minister was from a religious party regarded by some observers as conservative, so they were apprehensive as to whether she would support abortion rights or not.

In November 2000 activists were shocked by the news that one of their colleagues, Dr Sarsanto Sarwono, had been arrested at his clinic on charges of carrying out abortions. It had been unheard of previously for the police to arrest a doctor on such charges without evidence of harm to a patient or complaint from an irate spouse. It was also unusual for police to target a person with strong personal connections. Sarsanto is the son of two of the pioneers of the Indonesian family planning movement, and was well known as an officer of national professional medical associations. As he sat in the police station patiently answering the vague questions being put by arresting officers, his interrogators became more unsettled by the string of professors, civil servants, activists and former patients who came demanding to know what was going on. Clearly the police were caught in a situation they little understood.

Within days the matter was resolved. Somehow a disgruntled university colleague had motivated the police to arrest Sarsanto. The charge of abortion had nothing to do with the true complaint, and it took only a short time for senior police to see that their underlings had been used for frivolous purposes. The event mobilised the activist community, and found them making common cause with police, legal experts and key health officials. It was clear that the vagaries of the laws concerning abortion served no good purpose for women's health. As in the case of Suzanne Houtman seven decades earlier, the law had been used as an instrument of personal attack.

Within weeks the activists had revised their attitude towards abortion laws. Whereas before they had hoped to convince the Department of Health to ignore the strong anti-abortion language of the Criminal Code and the vague double talk of the 1992 Health Law, now they declared that nothing short of wholesale reform would protect patients and doctors from arbitrary interventions by the police and courts. They thus resolved to work with the legislature to amend the law. At the start of 2001 a coalition was formed including supporters from all major political parties and a key official from the Ministry of Health. By July this coalition had become the Indonesian Women's Health Foundation (*Yayasan Kesehatan Perempuan – YKP*), had raised money for a secretariat and had begun the task of drafting the clauses needed to redefine the position of abortion in the health law.

Laws in the New Order government had been drafted by individual government departments or ministries and passed on to the legislature for debate and endorsement. In the Reform Era, the legislative committee responsible for health matters (in 1999–2004 it was called Commission VII, becoming Commission IX in 2004–2009) decided to take the novel approach of drafting a law specifically on reproductive health to be presented to the government as both a challenge and a practical means of forcing positive change to the flawed 1992 law. Both legislators and activists were quickly advised that this could be a dangerous course of action since the bureaucracy retained substantial latent powers to distract or delay DPR initiatives.

In June 2002 the Minister of Health was approached privately and directly to elicit his support; he gave his blessing to the initiative and delegated the Director General for Community Health to assist. That person, though a long-time supporter of family planning, proved less than helpful in promoting the proposal. He said that the department had received threats from conservative religious leaders who were concerned about the moral implications of abortion. If it was easy to terminate a premarital pregnancy, they had argued, immorality would flourish. This was an argument he found hard to refute. The Ministry was finding that the Reform Era provided space for forces concerned with a variety of views on abortion, and officials were apt to try to satisfy all of them.

YKP replied that they would undertake research on the demand for abortion to show that most procedures were sought by married women whose contraceptive methods had failed. They could do this easily by examining the records of the largest network of abortion clinics in the country, the Indonesian Planned Parenthood Association (IPPA). Ironically, at that time the head of the Association was none other than the Director General who was warning them about the religious opposition and counselling them to drop the issue. He ordered the IPPA clinics not to participate in the research. As so often happens in the very small world of reproductive health activism in Indonesia, the YKP was closely connected to the doctors working for the IPPA. All the clinics adopted a policy of passive resistance. They said they would participate in the study but without using the IPPA name. The study went ahead and was published in 2004 (Widyantoro and Lestari).

While the researchers were in the field in 2002 the YKP staff went to the DPR to discuss the need for amendments to the Health law of 1992, in order to clarify the legal status of abortion. They met with Commission VII, the source of the original law, but now composed of a new group of motivated legislators keen to make a mark on the health system. They immediately put the amendment of the health law on to their agenda. Discussions dragged on for two years. In the end, as the parliament reached the end of their term, there was agreement that the abortion amendment should be very simple as set out here in Document 8.1.

Document 8.1. 2004 Indonesian Draft Amendment to Health Law 23/1992, Article 80

Article 80

(1) Government is obliged to prevent, protect and save a woman's lives from unsafe and irresponsible abortion practices through applicable laws and regulations.

(2) Unsafe abortion practices, as stated in paragraph (1), includes procedures:

a. Performed with force and without the consent of the woman;
b. Performed by unskilled health workers;
c. Performed without the application of professional standards; or
d. Performed in a discriminatory fashion or prioritising the fees charged rather than the welfare of women.

In February 2004, all political parties signed a Letter of Agreement supporting the draft law including the abortion amendment (YKP, 2004) and the matter was sent to the full DPR for confirmation. Soon, though, the DPR was distracted by the elections held in April 2004 under which all seats were up for grabs. The entire nation became mesmerised by the 'festival' of democracy as, in short order, new DPR members would take their seats. Then in July the first round for the first direct election of the President was carried out. As incumbent Megawati failed to gain an absolute majority in the first round, the election was required to go to a second round. Megawati faced a challenge from former general Susilo Bambang Yudhoyono, a formidable opponent whose promises were appealing to the electorate.

In August 2004, the draft amendment of the Health Law was still sitting on the desk of President Megawati. She called in members of YKP to have lunch with her and to discuss the implications of the legal change. They stressed the realities of women's health conditions and explained the confusion that had arisen concerning the legal status of abortion. The President said she would sign the law. But in order to follow proper procedure she would first need a letter from the Minister of Health supporting the amendment, particularly since she was in something of a lame duck position following the first round of election results.

The second round of voting took place on 24 September and Susilo Bambang Yudhoyono won by a substantial margin. When he was sworn in on 24 October 2004, the draft amendment had not been signed by Megawati and thus it expired. There had been no letter from the minister, despite many reminders from the YKP. Rumour had it that the task of drafting a comment had gone down into the bowels of the organisation where an anti-abortion official ensured that it could not be completed. Whether true or apocryphal, the result was the same: YKP and the network of reproductive health advocates were back to square one. The amendment would have to make its way through the DPR again.

The new legislature included many more rigid people from religious oriented parties than the previous DPR. Also many of the strong supporters of health reform had failed in their election attempts or had retired. In August 2005, the nature of the debate shifted. The *Hizbut Tahir* Islamic group sent a message calling on the President to put a stop to any proposal to legalise abortion in any form. They linked the call to their campaign to promote *Syariah* law across the country, and claimed to have sent 'a million' messages to the President's SMS address. While they are only a very small political group, they were able to command public attention through application of communications technologies and recruitment of sympathetic journalists. This changed the emotional tone of the debate. A newspaper article from that time captures the feeling:

> **The Masses of HTI Reject the Legalization of Abortion.**
>
> Hundreds of supporters of Hisbut Tahrir Indonesia (HTI) carried out coordinated protests across a number of cities... The issue that they raised is the rejection of legalised abortion, that is the amendment of the Health Law of 1992. A spokesman for the protesters, Muhammad Riyan said that before the legalization of abortion the government had to resolve the question of why there is any demand for

> abortion. First, legalization of abortion cannot be regarded as a solution to the problems of maternal mortality and unwanted pregnancy. Second, even if abortion is allowed under [some interpretations of] Islam, it can only be done to save the life of the mother and can only be allowed before 'ensoulment'. Third, unregulated legalization of abortion will only serve to increase the number of people offering abortion services. Fourth, HTI strongly rejects efforts at legalizing abortion such as those found in the draft amendment of the Health Law. Only by a return to Islamic systems of law will all these issues be resolved. (www.depkes.go.id/index.php?option=news&task=view article&sid=1244&Itemid=2)

Despite the strong language of this attack, and the attempt to organise street protests and SMS 'attacks' on the mobile phones of activists, the HTI group carried little force in the parliament. Nonetheless, when the amendment was discussed in the newly formed Komisi IX DPR committee for Population, Health, Labour Force and Transmigration, it was totally revised with many negative references to abortion as a concept, and complex language surrounding conditions under which women might obtain abortions from trained medical staff. Examples of this language, found in the draft, are shown in Appendix 8.2.

If history is any guide, the outcome of passing such an amendment will be a contradictory mixture of values, rules and moral declarations that will do little to provide legal surety to either doctors or the women seeking to terminate unwanted pregnancies. As a result, women will continue to rely on ambiguity and secrecy to provide options for their reproductive health.

People are afraid to be seen opposing statements of religious leaders even if they defy them in their private behaviour. There is a huge element of self-deceit that has been reinforced by three decades of 'rigid official' religiosity. This has been translated into grass-roots movements in favour of Islamic legal practices that would control women's behaviour and particularly the behaviour of the unmarried. Some groups teach that family planning is evil. Women are made to feel that they are 'unfaithful' to their husbands if they decide to adopt a contraceptive or have an abortion without his permission. While this may indeed reflect the preferences of some women, the problem is that such ideas are being translated into law by members of conservative religious movements.

Even as the Health Law was being debated, the draft Law on Population that had been working its way through the DPR for six years was still mired in committee discussions and interdepartmental rivalry. Originally focussed on family planning, over the years it gained sections dealing with vital registration, migration and labour force. Anti-abortion fundamentalists in the DPR in 2007 added clauses concerning abortion to the mix. It is uncertain if the law will ever pass and be submitted to the President, but if it did, it would mean that Indonesia could have three contradictory laws concerning the termination of pregnancy. The Health Minister in the 2004–9 Cabinet came from a Muhammadiyah background and encouraged YKP to obtain a reform of the law. The reformers included many strong Islamic groups including Rahima and the Fatayat Nahdlatul Ulama. However, nothing is easy in the Indonesian legal jungle and it remains unclear what will emerge. Parliamentary elections in April 2009 produced a new line up with fewer religious fundamentalists and more women, but the lack of clear party policies or publicly announced ideologies means that it is always difficult to predict how the parliamentary committees will behave.

Conclusion

Two centuries of legal arguments over abortion have not clarified Indonesian women's reproductive rights. They continue to die due to unsafe abortions. Unwanted pregnancies continue to place women in highly disadvantageous social dilemmas. If students become pregnant, they are expelled from schools. If workers experience a contraceptive failure, they face the unenviable choice of leaving their job or having an illegal pregnancy termination. Poor couples attempting to limit their family size are denied the option of safe abortion in a cultural context that condemns the practice. Medical practitioners and patients face vague but emotional moral declarations from other community members. The political culture of the bureaucracy remains hierarchical, authoritarian and mechanistic, producing high levels of corruption. It is in this context that over one million women obtain abortions each year in Indonesia, with no guarantee of safety. It is impossible to obtain accurate data on either the number of abortions or the harm caused by unsafe practices. The Ministries of Health and Women's Empowerment are unable to provide data on the numbers of unlicensed practitioners arrested, charged or convicted under the different laws regulating abortion. Despite a huge industry of traditional medicine claiming to bring on late periods there is no information about the use of these concoctions or the impact they have to either terminate a pregnancy (through the induction of menses) or alternatively the impact they have on a foetus exposed to these materials. What is clear though is that women are disadvantaged by the lack of clarity in the law.

In one hundred and fifty years, abortion technology has improved to the point where it is one of the safest medical procedures available. Social changes in the twentieth century have produced greater education, higher employment and greater pressure for gender equality. For Indonesian feminists, all these changes appear to be a mirage – safe abortion appears within reach, but continues to disappear just as they seem to reach their goals. The politics of abortion law reform and arguments over reproductive moralities remain major barriers and women continue to suffer.

Acknowledgments

Thanks to colleagues who have helped us track down some of the hidden information about the history and politics of abortion in Indonesia, including: Dr Djayadilaga, Dr Kartono Mohamad, Members of the Indonesian Women's Health Foundation, Dr Meiwita Budiharsana, Dr Firman Lubis, Mrs Madelon Harlon, Dr Gerry van Klinken, and Dr David Henley. Thanks to Dr Valerie Hull for comments on an early draft of this paper.

Appendix

DOCUMENT 8.2 Translation of Indonesian Health Law No. 23/1992

Article 15

(1) In case of emergency, as an effort to save the life of the pregnant woman and or her foetus, 'certain medical procedures' (*tindakan medis tertentu*) can be performed.

(2) Certain medical procedures, as stated in paragraph (1), may only be performed if:

a. Based on medical indications the procedures are required;

b. [The procedure must be] performed by a health worker possessing the necessary skills and authority, under the guidance of an expert team;

(continued)

c. Under the consent of the pregnant woman or her husband or family;

d. Must be performed in a certain health-care facility.

(3) Other regulations on the subject of a certain medical actions, as stated in paragraph (1) is enacted under the government regulations.

Explanations of the paragraphs:

(1) Medical procedures in the form of 'abortion' (*pengguguran kandungan*), for any reason are forbidden because they violate legal norms, religious norms, ethical norms and norms of propriety. Nevertheless, in case of emergency, and with the purpose of saving the life of a pregnant woman and / or the foetus in her womb, it is permissible to carry out certain medical procedures.

(2) [Certain medical procedures referred to in Paragraph (1) can only be carried out if]:

a. A medical indication is a condition that truly requires a certain medical procedure to be carried out, because without the certain medical procedure the pregnant woman's and/or her foetus's life would be threatened.

b. Health workers allowed to carry out certain medical procedures are workers who have the skills and authority to do so, that is a specialist obstetrician-gynaecologist. Before carrying out certain medical procedures the health worker must request the approval of an expert team with members drawn from various fields such as medicine, religion, law and psychology.

c. The primary right to give consent [to certain medical procedures] rests with the pregnant woman herself except in cases where she is unconscious or otherwise unable to give her consent, in which case it can be given by her husband or her family.

d. Approved health facilities are those which possess adequate staff and equipment to carry out such medical procedures, and which are approved by the government

Document 8.3 2006 Indonesian Draft Health Law

Article 84

(1) All persons are prohibited from carrying out abortion.

(2) Prohibition, as stated in paragraph (1), may be excepted under the following circumstances:

a. Emergency medical indications detected during early pregnancy, which could harm the life of the mother and/or the

foetus may suffer from a fatal genetic illness and/or genetic retardation that cannot be cured and may threaten (*menyulitkan*) the life of the baby.
b. Emergency medical indication, on the subject that the foetus suffer from a fatal genetic illness and/or [severe] disability which cannot be cured, as stated in letter (a), must be performed with the consent of the mother and/or the father of the foetus.
c. Pregnancy due to rape that may cause psychologic trauma for a victim referred by an institution or by a local religious expert or leader according to the religious norms; and
d. Counselling and advice pre procedure and ended with counselling post procedure, performed by trained counsellor.

(3) Other regulations on the subject of emergency medical indication and rape, as stated in paragraph (2) letter (b) and letter (c), [will be] addressed by Ministerial Regulations.

Article 85

(1) Abortion, as stated in article 84, may only be performed, if:
a. it is carried out before the pregnancy reaches 6 weeks, counting from the first day of the last menstruation, except in case of medical emergency,
b. it is performed by a health worker possessing the necessary skills and authority, as certified by the Minister;
c. it is carried out with the consent of the pregnant woman;
d. it is carried out with the consent of the husband, except for victims of rape, and
e. it is performed in a health-care facility which meets conditions determined by the Minister.

Article 86 [based on the 2004 amendment]

(1) Government is obliged to protect women from inadequate, unsafe and irresponsible abortion practices, which also against the religion norms and the applicable laws and regulations.

(2) Inadequate, unsafe and irresponsible abortion practice includes practices:
a. Performed with force and without the consent of the woman;
b. Performed by unskilled health workers;
c. Performed without the standard of professions and services;
d. Performed with discrimination; or
e. Prioritising the fee charged by medical providers.

(3) Adequate, safe and responsible abortion should be performed based on the medical emergency indications determined by authorised health workers and advised by an institution or head or expert of a religious organization in accord with religious norms.

References

Anshor, M. U.. 2006. *Fikih Aborsi: Wacana Penguatan Hak Reproduksi Wanita.* Jakarta: Kompas Media Nusantara.

Asshiddiqie, J. 2006. *Perkembangan dan Konsolidasi Lembaga Negara Pasca Reformasi. [Institutional Development and Consolidation in the Post Reform State].* Jakarta: Konstitusi Press.

Dewi, M. H. U. 1997. *Aborsi Pro dan Kontra di Kalangan Petugas Kesehatan. [Abortion Pro and Contra Among Health Workers].* Yogyakarta: Pusat Penelitian Kependudukan UGM

Dixon-Mueller, R. 1993. *Population Policy and Women's Rights: Transforming Reproductive Choice.* Westport: Praeger.

Hawari, H. D.. 2006. *Aborsi: Dimensi Psikoreligi [Abortion: Psychoreligious Dimensions].* Jakarta: Faculty of Medicine, University of Indonesia.

Hull, T. H., N. Widyantoro and S. W. Sarwono. 2003. 'Induced Abortion in Indonesia.' *Studies in Family Planning.* 24 (4): 241–251.

Majelis Ulama Indonesia. 2005. Fatwa Tentang Aborsi (Determination Concerning Abortion) Number 4 of 2005. in H. Jurnalis Uddin et al. (eds), *Reinterpretasi Hukum Islam Tentang Aborsi.* Jakarta: Universitas Yarsi, pp. 271–280.

Mitra Inti Indonesia. 2005. *Temuan Terkini Upaya Penatalaksanaan Kehamilan Tak Direncanakan. Hasil Seminar Sehari [Initial findings of efforts to deal with unwanted pregnancies].* Proceedings of a one-day seminar held on 11 August 2004 at the Hilton Hotel. Jakarta: Mitra Inti Foundation.

Purwanto, E. A. and W. Kumorotomo. 2005. *Birokrasi Publik Dalam Sistem Politik Semi-Parlementar [Public Bureaucracy in a Quasi-parliamentary Political System].* Yogyakarta: Penerbit Gava Media.

Utomo, B. et al. 2001. *Incidence and Social-Psychological Aspects of Abortion in Indonesia: A Community-Based Survey in 10 Major Cities and 6 Districts, Year 2000.* Jakarta: Center for Health Research University of Indonesia.

Widyantoro, N. and H. Lestari, eds. 2004. *Laporan Penelitian Penghentian Kehamilan tak Diinginkan (KTD) Yang Aman Berbasis Konseling: Penelitian di 9 Kota Besar.* Jakarta: Yayasan Kesehatan Perempuan.

Yayasan Kesehatan Perempuan (YKP). 2004. *Kumpulan Makalah dan Tanggapan Fraksi-Fraksi DPR-RI Mengenai Perubahan Undang-Undang Nomor 23 Tahun 1992 Tentang Kesehatan [Collection of Papers and Opinions of Political Factions of the Indonesian Parliament Concerning Changes to Law Number 23 of 1992 on Health].* Jakarta: Women's Health Foundation.

Chapter Nine

Access to abortion services in Malaysia

A rights-based approach

Rashidah Abdullah and Yut-Lin Wong

Despite relatively liberal abortion laws in Malaysia, there are widespread misconceptions among Malaysians that abortion is illegal. Access to abortion services remains restricted in the public health care system. In contrast, expensive private-sector services, while widely available, cannot be accessed by low-income women. Disadvantaged women, such as those in violent relationships, poor women and unmarried women who have unwanted pregnancies experience difficulty accessing abortion despite their legal rights. In 2003, the incidence of abortion in Malaysia was reported as thirty-eight per one thousand women aged fifteen to forty-nine (Family Care International, 2003:4). However, due to the current legal and moral ambiguities surrounding abortion, data on incidence and prevalence patterns are not readily available.

The Penal Code Amendment Act (1989) allows a medical practitioner registered under the 1971 Medical Act to 'terminate the pregnancy of a woman if such medical practitioner is of the opinion, formed in good faith, that the continuance of the pregnancy would involve risk to the life of the pregnant women or injury to the mental and physical health of the pregnant woman greater than if the pregnancy were terminated' (Penal Code [Amendment Act] 1989,

Section 312). The former 1971 Penal Code Act only allowed abortion to save the life of the woman. The liberal conditions of the 1989 reform placed Malaysia on par with three-fifths of countries worldwide (WHO 2003). Unfortunately, this law reform was not widely publicised for fear that it may be misused (*The Star,* 1989) and was largely viewed as a reform by doctors to protect doctors. Many feminists, medical practitioners, NGOs and women in the general population have been unaware of the changes to the law and therefore access to the benefits of the law has been restricted. For example, a survey of 112 doctors and nurses from the state of Negri Sembilan in 2007 found that only 57 per cent correctly knew the law on termination of pregnancy and the others thought it was much more restricted (RRAAM 2007).

In the 1990s, the Malaysian government took the important policy step of recognising women's reproductive rights to decide on the children they wanted and to have high-quality services available following the declarations of the International Conference on Population and Development (ICPD) Programme of Action (1994; see Whittaker, this volume). The international policy documents of CEDAW, the Cairo ICPD Programme of Action, and the Beijing Women's conference were ratified by the government, providing a clear rights-based framework on women's health, reproductive health and reproductive rights. Following the Cairo and Beijing meetings, the government has used the term 'reproductive rights' in its documents and the reproductive health programme has been conceptualised as having ten components including legal abortion services. The government's stand, however, is that reproductive rights are for married couples only.

Almost fifteen years after the 1994 Cairo conference, however, 'reproductive rights' has not yet become a term that either women's groups, health providers or women themselves regularly use to advocate for women's entitlement to reproductive health services, including to accessible, affordable and quality contraception and abortion. There has been no significant progress in Malaysia in implementing the Cairo Programme of Action (ARROW, 2005). Population and family planning policy has remained low key and unclear, use of modern contraceptives is still low at 33.3 per cent and only slightly increased since 1984 (30 per cent), with overall contraceptive prevalence at 51.9 per cent (Huang, 2007). The Fourth Malaysian Population and Family Survey (MPFS-4) (2000) reported that 24.9 per cent of currently married women said they did not want any more children but were not using any contraceptive method.

The unmet need for married women aged twenty to twenty-four years was 20 per cent and that for those aged forty-five to forty-nine was about 42 per cent (Huang 2007).

Unmet need is confounded by the grave difficulty in accessing contraceptives. As discussed in this chapter, some of the health services' policies and practices regarding distribution of contraception contribute to access difficulties, including policies such as providing contraception only to married women and targeting them just after childbirth. Unmarried but sexually active women, as well as women who have stopped attending maternal care clinics thus miss out on services. Men are almost completely left out, as contraception is mainly promoted as part of maternal care services.

One of the biggest obstacles to implementation has been the lack of political interest and commitment to reproductive rights. For example, in 1996 a women's NGO suggested to the then Minister for Women, Family and Community Development that low contraceptive use was a critical women's health and reproductive rights issue. The minister rejected the issue stating that 'family planning is too politically sensitive'.[2] Malaysian women's NGOs and health NGOs hesitated until recently to take up women's access to abortion and contraceptive services as priority reproductive health and rights advocacy issues. It was thought that addressing these issues openly might lead to a backlash and subsequent restriction of services. The Reproductive Rights Advocacy Alliance Malaysia (RRAAM), formed in 2007, is committed to advocating for women's increased access to contraception and abortion services as a reproductive right and ensuring that women's voices are heard. This chapter presents a situational analysis of barriers to access to abortion services in Malaysia; but it also constitutes an intervention, as it is hoped the chapter will be useful for Malaysian women and their allies working towards improving access.

Islam and Abortion

Part of the sensitivity of abortion as an issue in Malaysia is the tension between religion and politics. As a multicultural country, Malaysia has diverse religions including Islam, Christianity, Buddhism, Sikh, and animist beliefs. Islam is the majority religion followed by Malays, who constitute 58 per cent of the population. The Islamic political party (PAS) holds the majority in one state. This collusion of politics and religion predisposes the state to intervene more readily in personal morality issues. Islamic law is not centrally controlled, as each state can independently enact legislation as well as issue *fatwah* (judgements). There are no state *syariah* laws on contraception and abortion but rather different *fatwah,* most of which are more than twenty years old. *Fatwah* are also issued from the National Fatwah Council, which can be used as guidance; however, these must be adopted by the state governments before they can be legally enforced (Centre For Reproductive Rights and ARROW 2005).

A national *fatwah* passed in 1981 permits temporary contraceptive use for a wide number of women's health, socio-economic, and family welfare reasons. Sterilisation is forbidden as a permanent method but is permissible when a pregnancy endangers the life of the woman or when a woman is unable to use other contraceptive methods. The general understanding and practice in the National Family Planning Programme is that Islam allows temporary contraception for health and welfare reasons, whereas sterilisation should only be done for health reasons. Abortion is permissible under Islam for health and welfare reasons before ensoulment, which is regarded as happening at the time of quickening or movement of the foetus when it is 120 days old. Globally, this is the predominant view in Muslim countries, a reassuring fact that needs to be made widely known in Malaysia (Hessini 2007). In 2002, the National Fatwah Committee issued a *fatwah* stating that abortion after 120 days of pregnancy is not permitted and is considered murder unless the woman's life is in danger or in cases of foetal impairment. However, the *fatwah* is reported not to have been publicised for fear that it may be misused. It is interesting to speculate why this *fatwah* suddenly appeared around the time of the advocacy work on a new abortion act (Centre for Reproductive Rights and ARROW, 2005, RRAAM 2007b).

There remains uncertainty among both the public and service providers regarding Islamic views on contraception and abortion, as there has been neither open discussion nor clear guidelines issued. This was expressed at several large dialogues and national seminars with doctors and gynaecologists in the late 1990s and in 2001. Many commented that the dialogues were extremely useful, as they were the first time that abortion was openly discussed with doctors and Muslim scholars (Sisters in Islam1998). No research on the knowledge and attitudes of doctors regarding Muslim *fatwah* has been done to date. In society generally, there has been a trend towards more conservative interpretations of Muslim positions over the last twenty years. This has happened along with increased conservatism on other issues such as women's dress, morality of unmarried young people and so forth, as part of the global increase in Muslim fundamentalism.

The government family planning programme has not corrected misconceptions and fears regarding the Islamic permissibility of contraception and abortion, even though it has been pointed out by women's groups that this is a key issue for Muslim women (Rashidah Abdullah 2000). Qualitative studies by Malaysian feminists, which asked women questions about contraception, abortion and Islam found that Muslim women believed Islam does not forbid family planning and were clear that as long as the foetus was not formed, family planning would not be forbidden. They incorrectly believed deliberately aborting a child is against Islam. They considered it forbidden for wives to secretly practice family planning without the knowledge or blessing of their husbands (Yut-Lin Wong 2003) even though there are views that this is allowed in certain circumstances. Further research is needed on both Muslim attitudes and those of Catholic doctors. The Catholic Church has a more restrictive position on contraception and abortion than Islam and was opposed to the proposed reform to have an independent abortion act in 2002. The Catholic doctors and lawyers associations spoke out strongly against further liberalisation of the law in the media and were influential in the proposal not being accepted (RRAAM, 2007).

Women's Understandings of Abortion

Malaysian women use various terminologies to refer to abortion depending on their ethnic group. These ethnically specific terminologies reflect the meanings of abortion in the various cultures, in contrast to technical terms used within the clinical setting or among health providers. Malay women refer to abortion as *cuci,* meaning to wash or to cleanse. Another term is *buang,* meaning to discard or remove. To Hokkien-speaking Chinese women, abortion is referred to as *sei gin na,* meaning to wash the child; and they may speak of their situation as delayed menses, *la sum bo lai,* meaning the 'dirty thing [menses] has not come'. Tamil-speaking Indian women speak also of delayed menstruation, *vayiru kaluvanum,* 'I need stomach washing, I have no period'. Similarly, English-speaking women may use the term 'washout' to mean abortion. In contrast, among health providers, nurses and doctors, the abbreviation MR (menstrual regulation) is written in clients' records to describe pregnancy termination (Siti Fathilah Kamaluddin, 1998:55). In some public hospitals, health providers tend to use the term 'termination of pregnancy' or TOP.

Regardless of ethnicity, Malaysian women describe abortion as a process of washing away something that is not wanted from their bodies rather than terminating or disrupting a pregnancy, with no reference to an embryo or foetus. They describe abortion in ambiguous terms, as a process which will restore delayed menses, to ensure the body functions normally again. Siti Fathilah Kamaluddin notes that these local ethnic terms reflect the lack of clear legal or social sanction of abortion in Malaysia and also reflect reluctance to reveal oneself as sexually active (Siti Fathilah Kamaluddin 1997:82; see also Whittaker, Belton, Hoban and Rashid, this volume). Such terms may also make the act of abortion more acceptable at a personal level for women as a necessary act of washing, cleansing or discarding something unwanted from their bodies, to regulate a normal body function of menstruation.

A qualitative study of the reproductive life histories of seventy-one women drawn from the three major ethnic groups, found many respondents resorted to traditional abortion methods to control their fertility, such as going to village midwives (*bidan kampong*) who perform induced abortions, or buying herbal abortifacients that are freely available via informal networks and from Chinese medicine shops (Raj et al. 1998). The study revealed that many rural Chinese women rely on a combination of barrier contraceptives and abortion both to space births and to achieve the desired number of children. According to the study, such pragmatism prevailed despite their mistaken belief that abortion is illegal, their expressed moral reservations over abortion, and its dangers to women's health. Many Chinese women who had had abortions spoke frankly and openly of abortion as the only alternative whenever contraception failed. Malay women in the study regarded abortion as a 'sin' and believed that it is permissible only for serious health reasons and generally disapproved the idea of pregnant unmarried women resorting to abortions. Notwithstanding these attitudes, all Malay women in the study knew about traditional abortion methods as well as herbal abortifacients learned from village midwives or other women in the community, although none of them admitted to ever having had an abortion. Knowledge and availability of traditional methods within the Malay community confirmed the researchers' hypothesis that Malay women underreported both attempted and realised abortions (Raj et al. 1998: 135–138).

Siti Fathilah Kamaluddin's (1998) study of thirty-nine urban women also revealed local understandings of pregnancy, particularly foetus formation, and its importance to women's decision-making on abortion. For Malay Muslim women in her study, pre-counselling services included the use of ultrasound visuals in which they could see the actual foetus size. For these women, these visuals confirmed that the pregnancy was just a 'clot of blood' (*ketul darah*) and hence termination was acceptable (*halal*) according to Islamic teaching since there had been no ensoulment of the foetus. Some women expressed that the degree of one's attachment towards the foetus would help in deciding on abortion or not. They said when they did not feel any attachment, it would be easy to terminate the pregnancy (*tak sayang lagi*); but they could not do so if they thought the foetus' 'heart is beating inside me'.

Religious beliefs impact on women's perception of abortion and often deter women from deciding to abort. In Siti Fathilah Kamaluddin's study, women of varied religions commonly expressed guilt as they believed their religion regarded abortion as murder or, 'what God has given you, you can't take it away'. Those whose religious beliefs prohibited abortion and yet had to undergo termination feared punishment from God, fearing that they would become infertile. The study found that the more in control and clear the women were about their decision to end the pregnancy, the calmer and more stoic they were after the abortion and the more rapid their recovery.

Reasons Why Women Terminate Pregnancies

Malaysian women seek terminations for a variety of reason, including medical and financial reasons, contraceptive failure, lack of access to contraception, and social reasons. Fathilah (1998) undertook a qualitative study of thirty-nine women (the majority married factory workers) who had terminated a pregnancy in an urban clinic. Apart from those aborting for medical reasons such as high blood pressure and diabetes, women explained they just could not afford to raise an additional child above their existing family size of two or three children. The high cost of childcare was singled out as among the serious financial barriers against raising a child in the city. Working-class women, especially those who are rural-urban migrants, have no extended families to fall back on for childcare and subsidised crèches at the workplace are very rare. Young and single women in the study did not know about contraception and could not easily access contraceptives, except condoms sold in supermarkets; hence, they resorted to abortion as a contraception method instead. On the other hand, among those who had access to contraceptives, some experienced methods failure or severe side effects, making contraceptives unappealing. The researcher noted that some women received incomplete information that could have led to accidental misuse of certain contraceptives; or health providers had not warned of the cumulative risk of pregnancy or contraceptive failure associated with long-time use of specific contraceptives. It has been reported in a national survey that methods failure is 5.4 per cent (Huang 2007). Social reasons for terminating pregnancy included unwanted pregnancies as a result of rape, or those that occurred to drug users, sex workers, and unmarried women (Siti Fathilah Kamaluddin 1998). Some married women sought abortions because they or their husbands were unwilling to have a child, or because their husbands were having affairs, or because the pregnancies resulted from women's extramarital affairs. Women also reported unplanned pregnancies occurring because their husbands were opposed to contraceptives and the latest national demographic survey reported 12.5 per cent of married women did not use contraceptives because of their husband's objection (Huang 2007). A few Chinese women explained that since they were second wives or mistresses, not legal wives, their children would have no inheritance rights and hence they did not want to bear children but they had not used any contraceptives (Siti Fathilah Kamaluddin 1998).

Violence against women

A number of chapters in this book highlight the links between gender inequality, violence against women and abortion (see Belton, Whittaker). Anecdotal evidence from the Women's Aid Organisation (WAO) refuge suggests that a number of survivors of domestic violence experience abortions. According to Shoba Aiyar, Social Work Manager at WAO, an average of 120 battered women take shelter at WAO per year; half of them knew about and used contraceptives and the other half did not. Women reported between one to eight abortions, and one woman had experienced three recurrent abortions (Aiyar 2007). Women reported that having an abortion in a private clinic could cost between RM 300 (for first month of pregnancy) to RM 2,000 (for second trimester pregnancy; US$1= 3.4 Malaysian Ringgit). Although in a few cases the husbands paid for the abortions, the majority of women said it was difficult for them to secure the money required and were forced to sell or pawn their jewellery or beg the doctor to reduce the cost. A number experienced bleeding or complications resulting from incomplete abortion and were then forced to seek treatment in government hospitals.

Women within violent relationships spoke of complex power relations and counter negotiations between themselves and their partners. For such women, access to quality-care abortion services is even more critical and needs to be understood within this context of violence. Survivors of domestic violence explained that their violent husbands often forced sex on them, resulting in unwanted pregnancies. Half of the women who took refuge at WAO reported that their violent husbands forbid them to practice contraception. According to them, their husbands did not allow contraception so as to ensure their wives would not have sex with other men; husbands would also say sex is not pleasurable if a condom is used. Others wanted to impregnate their wives as often as possible so that other men would not find them attractive (this was especially the case if the wives were much younger). A few of the women deliberately did not use contraceptives so as to force their husbands to use condoms and would use the absence of a condom as a strategy to reject sex with their husbands. One woman who had had three recurrent abortions stated that getting pregnant was the only time she could get her husband's attention, although invariably he would want her to go for an abortion.

Violence against women underscores the impact of gender inequality that denies women the power to decide on childbearing and spacing. Consequently, women bear the burden of unplanned or unwanted pregnancies while men ignore their reproductive responsibilities.

Unmarried women and girls

The WAO also shelters unwed pregnant women and girls who have come to seek refuge. Their plight highlights the lack of sexual and reproductive health services for unmarried women and girls. Many of the unwed pregnant women and girls at the refuge became pregnant as a result of rape or coercion into sexual relations by boyfriends they thought would be their husbands one day. Instead, once pregnant, these boyfriends suggested abortions, or just abandoned them. These unwed pregnant women and girls were left to deal with the pregnancy themselves, sometimes with the help of friends and only rarely with help from their parents. By the time they managed to seek shelter at WAO, many were already in the third trimester of pregnancy and allowed WAO to arrange the adoption of their babies after delivery following legal procedures in liaison with government authorities. In a focus group discussion at WAO, these unwed pregnant women and girls recounted how they had been informed about pregnancy and family planning during secondary schooling, but had only felt it would be an issue after they got married and had children. They wished they could have had ready access to government health services and information on the options available to them. Instead, they were getting incorrect information on the legality of termination of pregnancy and did not know where to go for such procedures. Many of them confided that they had tried to abort by taking a variety of concoctions such as Panadol (paracetamol) plus Coke soft drink, raw papaya and pineapple, and even Clorox (a bleaching agent). Many suggested that if they had had access to proper health services and had had an abortion they would have experienced less stress than carrying their pregnancies to term and arranging for adoption (Aiyar, 2007).

The same vulnerabilities and lack of access to appropriate health services were common experiences in other studies of other unwed pregnant women and girls. Sexual coercion and the need to have sex with their boyfriends to prove their love were common themes. Having sex symbolises ownership by the boyfriend, something viewed as desirable; and some young women regarded having sex with their boyfriends as a way to repay him for his kindness and gifts or in return for payment of mobile phone bills and other items. As in other parts of Asia (see Whittaker 2004), local newspapers find it especially shocking that a good proportion of unwed pregnant women are educated university graduates or undergraduate students in local universities. One centre for women and teenagers run by a Muslim couple in the city was reported to provide shelter to eighty to one hundred unwed pregnant women and girls in a year, with about 40 per cent of them being undergraduates (*The New Paper* 2004). Likewise, reports of abandoned babies, seen as an indicator of unwed pregnancies, is regarded by the Malaysian press as a social ill infecting wayward youth. It has been reported that one baby is abandoned every ten days in Kuala Lumpur, the country's largest urban metropolis. From 2001 to 2004, the Welfare Department recorded 315 cases of abandoned babies, while police statistics revealed about one hundred cases a year (Ang 2007). Instead of a moral panic, there is an urgent need to address the lack of functional knowledge of sexual reproductive matters as well as the absence of related services for youth. According to the National Population and Family Development Board, a session held for secondary school students highlighted the findings of their Malaysian Population and Family Survey–4 that adolescents have little knowledge about their reproductive organs and their functions. Although only 2.4 per cent admitted to having had sex, 20.7 per cent of them said they knew of friends who had premarital sex; 21.2 per cent knew of friends who had illegitimate pregnancies and 10 per cent had friends who had had an abortion (*STAR* 2007). When young women are denied access or only have restricted access to abortion services, consequences range from the complications of incomplete abortion, even death, mental health problems and in some cases suicide, loss of opportunities to further one's career, being expelled from school, or loss of higher educational opportunities. Unmarried young women and girls in many countries are found to be willing to risk death or injury from unsafe abortion or use abortifacients rather than to give birth to unwanted babies (Hord 2001).

Barriers to Accessibility to Abortion Services in Hospitals

Women's access to legal abortions is being restricted by health providers' personal interpretations as well as unofficial policy and practice in the Ministry of Health. As Chee Heng Leng and Yut-Lin Wong note, the decision making power has been removed from individual women in favour of professionals (2007: 148). Given that the specific circumstances involved in 'injurious to physical and mental health' are not spelled out in the law, this depends on the individual doctors' interpretation. For the public sector, there is no written national Ministry of Health policy restricting abortion services; practice depends on the individual views of the Head of the Obstetrics and Gynaecology Department. Abortion services therefore do not appear to be regarded in public hospitals as a necessary and regular service in the package of reproductive health services provided to women. In some government hospitals, doctors who perform legal abortions are reported to be stigmatised and face difficulties regarding promotion (RRAAM 2007).

Since 2001, public hospitals follow standardised procedures, which state that abortion requests can be for medical and *psychiatric* reasons and requires doctors to obtain a second medical opinion. The doctor deciding on the abortion is not allowed to be the one who does the abortion. Counselling is also required involving a psychiatrist, medical social worker and doctors before a decision is made and after the abortion (Centre for Reproductive Rights and ARROW 2005). Clearly such procedures impose a number of delays to women's access to abortions and the legal conditions for abortion have been incorrectly stated and restricted to medical and *psychiatric* conditions, whereas the law states physical and the broader category of *mental health* reasons. It is thus difficult for a woman wanting an abortion and legally entitled to one, to have good access to abortion in public hospitals, given the current anti-abortion environment and the fact that doctors are being guided by these procedures. The procedures are much more complex than required by the law, which allows one doctor to make his or her assessment on the mental health of the woman. Under these procedures, a woman's access depends on the opinions of two doctors on whether or not the reasons are justifiable, as well as on the woman's ability to communicate and negotiate her needs and rights. For example, one public hospital's practice is to routinely obtain the psychiatrist's clearance, in addition to that of an obstetrician and gynaecologist; the psychiatrist is known to give clearance only to women who have shown signs of attempted suicide. Pre-abortion counselling is always done with both the woman and her husband to pre-empt subsequent litigation issues, whether or not the woman wants her husband to know; and the husband's signature is always required.

Case studies of the actual provision of abortion services in public hospitals, according to the law, reveal restricted accessibility. In the Klang Valley and in Negri Sembilan state, two hundred kilometres south of the capital, anecdotal evidence from doctors and lecturers is that abortion is done only in limited cases and not for the broad permissible legal reasons of possible injury to women's physical and mental health. Government doctors who do not do abortions refer women to private clinics. In one Kuala Lumpur hospital, an extreme reluctance to perform any kind of legal abortion was reported. Women whose foetuses were known to be grossly deformed were referred to other government hospitals in which there are doctors who are more comfortable with doing abortions. In another hospital, discussion of abortion among staff is not encouraged, raped women who want an abortion have difficulty getting access and hospital social workers are not allowed to provide referral services to the private sector for women seeking an abortion (RRAAM 2007).

Certain groups of women face even greater difficulties obtaining legal abortions from government hospitals. Unsympathetic and stereotyped views of women have become the norm in some hospitals without the realisation of the impact this has on women's choices and women's rights. There is evidence that unsympathetic judgements are formed on the morality of unmarried women's pregnancies and what is best for women who have been raped. These unsympathetic attitudes act as a service obstacle. A doctor from a government hospital in a rural state explained in the 2006 ARROW–FIGO Forum that her unwritten hospital policy and practice for raped pregnant women was to encourage them not to terminate the pregnancy but to give birth, as there were many couples waiting for babies to adopt (ARROW 2006). This attitude is verified by the 2007 survey of doctors and nurses in a southern state, which found that in response to the question, 'What do you think women who are pregnant due to rape should consider doing?' 38 per cent said that they should have the baby and either look after it themselves or give it up for adoption rather than consider having an abortion (RRAAM 2007).

Dilation and curettage (D&C) remains the predominant method used in government hospitals which requires anaesthetics and in-patient care and carries greater risks than vacuum aspirations. Due to high operating theatre demands, and the low priority of women waiting for the procedure, women doing D&C are reported to have longer waiting times than other patients (Rashidah Abdullah 2007). Medication abortion methods such as cytotec and mifepristone are not available in government hospitals. Women therefore have very limited choices on abortion methods. An encouraging advance is the establishment of Early Pregnancy Assessment Units, which can provide quicker, safer and cheaper vacuum aspiration methods as an outpatient service for miscarriages and abortion. The national network of Family Planning Association clinics do not provide abortion services but can refer women to doctors who do so. Four of the thirteen FPAs report providing regular referral. FFPAM and the FPAs do not yet have a policy requiring referral for abortion on a women's request nor on pre- and post-abortion services (RRAAM 2007).

Legal abortion services are reported to be widely available in the private sector in all private hospitals and in medical centres with gynaecological services. A few general practitioners also provide services however it is not known what types of abortions are available, nor the predominant methods used. The main issues regarding accessibility to private-sector services are that women do not know which clinics provide abortion services and what the associated costs are. Abortion services are not advertised; however, menstrual regulation for other purposes sometimes is. Women coming for services to *Kelinik Rakyat* in Penang (RRAAM 2007) and to WAO (Aiyar 2007) have reported that they had sought abortion in other clinics previously but could not afford the charges (which, as noted previously, ranged from RM 300 to RM 2,000). A fair fee for early abortion (which still gives a profit to the practitioner) is assessed to be RM 250. High fees are severely restricting poorer women's access to a safe abortion.

No known public-sector quality of care studies have been conducted which include asking women about their experiences and the extent of their satisfaction with the range of abortion services offered, beginning with pre-abortion counselling and ending with post-abortion care. Siti Fathilah Kamaluddin's (1998) women-centred research in an urban private clinic in Penang is the only such research and involves only one clinic. She found that women who have had an abortion come back to the same clinic for repeated abortions, despite the clinic's focus on contraceptive education. Her study recommended more innovative audiovisual education on contraception during post-abortion counselling for women at the clinic. Quality of pre-abortion counselling largely depends on the quality of training in counselling techniques and contraception education, the quality of service guidelines, monitoring and supervision and the time available and allocated for this service. It is not known if there are clear protocols and if these are well implemented. Recent discussions between providers in both the public and private sector have agreed that there is a need for more attention to, and training for, these aspects of abortion services (Hospital Tuanku Jaafar 2007).

Hence, women's access to *quality-care* abortion services is severely restricted by the prevalent misconception about legalities of abortion despite the relatively permissive abortion laws that exist. Due to the dire lack of a systematic data base on abortion incidence and prevalence in the country, a comprehensive understanding of the variations in women's access by socio-demographic factors is regrettably unavailable. However, the preceding discussion, based on available evidence, has pointed to the diverse and complex barriers affecting different categories of Malaysian women. Yet, it can be said that the misconception and misinterpretation of abortion laws impacts on access to quality-care abortion services by *all* women in the country, be they rich or poor, living in urban or rural areas. Misconception of abortion laws has resulted in the need for secrecy, lack of medical support, the risk of exposure and fear of imprisonment for both health providers and women seeking abortion. Such an environment encourages abortions to be carried out by clandestine and unskilled providers who operate in situations that endanger women's lives (J Ravindran 2003).

Advocacy: The Way Forward

Malaysia is fortunate in that the actual policies and laws on contraception and abortion are reasonable and do not require immediate reform in order to increase service access. Rather, the agenda is to increase the actual commitment, understanding and implementation of policy and law into services and training. A women's rights–based approach to advocacy is essential and must include documentation of women's experiences and violations of their rights. RRAAM (2007b) developed a list of indicators of the specific changes for advocacy (see Appendix 9.1). This requires strategic alliances and for the women's movement and other social movements to support these issues more strongly in their own advocacy agendas. In particular, it requires the medical, obstetrics and gynaecology and medico-legal associations to commit to women's issues of access and rights to legal abortion services.

In Malaysia, both government and private women's health services need to move towards operating according to a reproductive rights–based framework, which sees abortion services provided according to the law without stigma and judgement to women and adolescent girls, regardless of marital status. Government and private-sector service protocols on abortion need to clearly specify the situations in which a woman with an unwanted pregnancy is legally entitled to an abortion – such as cases of rape, incest, domestic violence, diseases and medical conditions worsened by the pregnancy, and mental health problems such as severe stress, anxiety, and depression and not only a psychiatric disorder, as is currently the case (cf. the situation in Thailand, Boonthai et al. this volume). The woman concerned should be the one to define the effect an unwanted pregnancy has on her mental health, as she is the one to go through pregnancy and rear the child. Clinics unable to provide full abortion services should provide comprehensive referral services to women who request an abortion. Requirements for consent of spouses and parents for abortion, sterilisation and childbirth should be removed, where legally possible, to recognise women's reproductive rights. WHO best practice guidelines for terminations need implementation, with menstrual regulation/vacuum aspiration provided to women as the safest and cheapest method in early pregnancy. The full range of methods of abortion, including medical abortion, should be made available to women.

To prevent unwanted pregnancies and abortion, Malaysia needs to improve the uptake of modern contraceptive methods. All the methods of contraception need to be easily available and affordable, in public and private health services, including male and female sterilisation, female condoms and diaphragms. Service providers and the media need to develop more creative and effective means to increase the use of male methods of contraception and to increase men's support for contraception and abortion. As part of this, emergency contraception needs to be available (and be made known to be available) in all public and private hospitals, clinics and pharmacies so as to prevent unwanted pregnancy and abortion. Improved contraceptive education and provision is required as part of pre- and post-abortion counselling.

RRAAM will continue to engage with media services to provide more accurate information to women and the public on contraception and abortion. We hope to make all RRAAM information easily available on websites and in our publications, including the latest research findings, women's experiences; best practices in contraceptive and abortion services with tools and checklists for pre- and post-abortion counselling. In particular, medical and nursing curricula in public and private educational institutions need to be amended to include comprehensive contraceptive and abortion content, including training in carrying out sterilisation and abortion methods. Similarly, it needs to be determined why recommendations made over the last thirty years for comprehensive sexuality and reproductive health information education to be implemented by schools, in the media and on websites for young people have not been achieved.

The final part of RRAAM's recommendations advocates for more women-centred research and evidence. This includes a comprehensive plan for priority research on contraception and abortion access by academics, government and NGOs addressing the main barriers and identified gaps in knowledge. More documentation of women's stories of abortion and contraception need to be collected as evidence of access issues, women's unmet needs and violations of women's reproductive rights. Similarly, the disaggregation of government health system data on contraception and abortion by age, race, income, education and location is required in order to guide program and service provision.

Based on our situational analysis, it is clear that in Malaysia abortion is permitted by law but is commonly unavailable or inaccessible. Rights-based sexual reproductive health services would mainstream abortion services into the health system, with simple protocols, so as to make access easy. Compared to the currently stigmatised and clandestine practice, women should be able to legally terminate pregnancy safely, openly and affordably.

Our advocacy is producing encouraging progress. The Ministry of Health (MOH) has responded positively to the advocacy efforts of RRAAM targeted at health care providers. During 2007–2008, RRAAM presented evidence on the poor knowledge of doctors on the abortion law, their misconceptions and unsympathetic attitudes to rape and unplanned pregnancies and engaged the MOH in dialogue (FRHAM and RRAAM 2009a,b). The MOH is now working on service guidelines for doctors in government clinics and hospitals so that abortion services will be more accessible. In 2009, the MOH partnered with RRAAM in holding two state-level seminars attended by a total of 220 doctors and nurses from both the public and private sectors aimed to educate on the law, women-centred abortion services, reproductive rights and ethical issues. The MOH will continue to partner with RRAAM in organizing such advocacy seminars for health care providers to cover all thirteen Malaysian states. Meanwhile, for the first time, the Obstetrical and Gynaecological Society of Malaysia (OGSM) has openly discussed abortion law, services and access issues in the Nineteenth Annual Congress, 2009, in a symposium on reproductive rights in which RRAAM was invited to speak on these issues.

Such positive responses and actions from the MOH and OGSM constitute substantive progress. This shows that strategic advocacy on abortion can be effective especially when initiated by a committed multi-sectoral alliance of feminist researchers, NGO activists, rights- and gender-oriented doctors, lawyers and national network of reproductive health associations.

Notes

1. Study of the Kelantan Family Planning Association (KFPA) new clients' clinic record card including abortion incidence by one of authors who was state organiser of KFPA for four years from 1975 to 1999.
2. Discussion with the said Minister at Sisters in Islam office in 1996 by one of the authors.

Appendix 9.1
The Reproductive Rights Advocacy Alliance Malaysia (RRAAM) advocacy outcome indicators.

COMMITTED and EFFECTIVE ADVOCACY

- The Reproductive Rights Advocacy Alliance Malaysia [RRAAM] becomes stronger with more influential allies, and succeeds in helping to bring about concrete changes in contraception and abortion services availability, accessibility, affordability and quality.
- Medical, Obstetrics and Gynaecology, and Medico Legal Associations extend their advocacy agenda from protection of doctors to commit to women's issues of access and rights to legal abortion services.
- The women's movement and other social movements support these issues more strongly in their own advocacy agenda and in solidarity with RRAAM.

OPEN and ACCURATE INFORMATION and EDUCATION

- Understanding, compassion and openness to women's diverse needs for abortion and their legal and reproductive rights greatly increases among service providers, the media, the public and policy makers due to new women-centred evidence.
- An urgent NGO and human rights enquiry is undertaken to determine why recommendations and plans for 30 years for comprehensive sexuality and reproductive health information education to be implemented in schools, the media and websites for young people has not been achieved and the way forward.
- High quality information is easily available on websites and in publications on all RRAAM issues including the law and policy; the latest research including women's experiences; best practices in contraceptive and abortion services with tools and checklists for pre- and post-abortion counselling.
- The media regularly engage with RRAAM and its allies for dialogue and information and provide more accurate and responsible information to women and the public on contraception and abortion.
- Medical and nursing curricula in public and private educational institutions are amended to include comprehensive contraceptive and abortion content including training in carrying out sterilization and abortion methods.

BETTER WOMEN-CENTRED RESEARCH and EVIDENCE

- Increased recognition by policy makers, service providers and the media that effective contraceptive use is low for a developed country like Malaysia and that family planning services need to be urgently strengthened for better prevention of unwanted pregnancies and abortion due to non contraceptive use.

- A comprehensive plan for priority research on contraception and abortion access by academics, government and NGOs addressing the main barriers [attitude, knowledge, policy, service practice etc] is drawn up based on identified gaps and the need for new knowledge.
- More documented women's stories/experiences on abortion and contraception as evidence of access issues, women's needs and violations of reproductive rights issues are collected, presented to and discussed by policy makers and service providers.
- Data on contraception and abortion are disaggregated by age, race, income, education, and location are routinely collated by the government health system and are widely available to guide programmes.

WOMEN'S HEALTH SERVICES HAVE A WOMEN-CENTRED AND REPRODUCTIVE RIGHTS-BASED FRAMEWORK

- Abortion services according to the law are routinely provided without stigma and judgment to women and adolescent girls as a basic reproductive health service in the package of reproductive health services in the MOH hospitals and clinics.
- MOH and private sector service protocols on abortion specify the very clear situations in which a woman with an unwanted pregnancy is legally entitled to an abortion – eg. rape, incest, domestic violence, diseases and medical conditions worsened by the pregnancy, mental health problems [severe stress, anxiety, depression and not only a psychiatric disorder].
- A reproductive rights approach is taken to abortion services and sterilisation that it is the woman who defines the effect an unwanted pregnancy has/will have on the state of her mental health is the main decision maker, as she is the one to go through pregnancy and rear the child.
- MOH, FPA, GP Clinics and women NGO crisis services who are not able to provide full abortion services, follow protocols to provide comprehensive referral services to women who request an abortion [without any assessment or judgement], using a reliable list of public hospitals or private clinics known to provide the services.
- Emergency contraception is available [and known to be available] in all public hospitals and clinics [including district hospitals and private clinics] for rape and incest cases and for other clear emergencies so as to prevent unwanted pregnancy and abortion.
- Contraceptive education and provision is given increased time as part of pre and post abortion counselling so as to better prevent further abortions due to incorrect and non-use of contraceptives.
- Increased efforts of service providers and media to reach out more creatively and effectively to men so as to increase use of male methods and men's support for contraception and abortion.

- All the methods of contraception are easily available and affordable for women's choice, in public and private health services, including male and female sterilization, female condoms and diaphragms.
- Requirements for consent of spouses and parents for abortion, sterilization and childbirth are removed where legally possible in recognition of the need to have no gatekeepers to women's reproductive rights and in respect of confidentiality.
- All the methods of abortion are available for women and adolescent girls to choose from, and menstrual regulation/vacuum aspiration is explained as the safest and cheapest method in early pregnancy.
- Private sector clinics reduce the fees for abortion and/or have a sliding scale according to income. Cheaper and safer menstrual regulation is the main method provided for early abortion.

Source: RRAAM 2007b

References

Ang, E. S. 2007. 'Adolescent Health', *National Population Conference 3–5 July 2007.* Kuala Lumpur.

ARROW. 2005. *Monitoring Ten Years of ICPD Implementation. The Way Forward. Asian Country Reports.* Kuala Lumpur: ARROW.

———. 2006. *ARROW–FIGO Parallel Forums on Sexual and Reproductive Health and Rights,* November 2006. Kuala Lumpur: ARROW.

Centre for Reproductive Rights and ARROW. 2005. Malaysia. *Women of the World: Laws and Policies Affecting Their Reproductive Lives. East and South East Asia.* New York: Centre For Reproductive Rights.

Chee, H. L. and Y. L. Wong. 2007. 'Women's access to health care services in Malaysia', in H. L. Chee and S. Barraclough (eds), *Health Care in Malaysia: the dynamics of provision, financing and access.* London: Routledge, pp. 137–153.

Family Care International. 2005. 'Saving Women's Lives: The Health Impact of Unsafe Abortion', *Report of a Conference held in Kuala Lumpur, Malaysia, 29 September – 2 October 2003.* Geneva: WHO.

FRHAM and RRAAM. 2009a. 'Report on High-Level GO-NGO ICPD15 Policy Dialogue: Increasing Access to the Reproductive Right to Contraceptive Information and Services, SRHR Education for Youth and Legal Abortion', 27 May 2009, Subang Jaya, Selangor: FRHAM and RRAAM.

———. 2009b. 'ICPD 15 Monitoring and Advocacy on Sexual and Reproductive Health and Rights [SRHR]: Unwanted Pregnancies, The Critical SRHR Issues of Low Contraceptive Use, Lack of Sexual and Reproductive Health Education for Youth and Accessibility to Legal Abortion - Malaysia Country Report', 7 July 2009, Kuala Lumpur:

Hessini, L. 2007. 'Abortion and Islam: Policies and Practice in the Middle East and North Africa', *Reproductive Health Matters* 15 (29): 75–84.

Hord, C. E. 2001. *Making safe abortion accessible: A practical guide for advocates.* Chapel Hill, NC: Ipas.

Huang, M. 2007. 'Prevention: Increasing Contraceptive Use', *Seminar on Reproductive Health, Rights and Miscarriages: Problems & Solutions, 3 July 2007.* Hospital Tuanku Ja'afar, Seremban, Negeri Sembilan, Malaysia.

Penal Code No574, 312[1997] [Malay] amended by Penal Code [Amendment] Act No 727 [1989].

J. Ravindran, 2003. 'Unwanted Pregnancy: Medical and Ethical Dimensions', *Medical Journal of Malaysia* 58 Supplement A: 23–35.

Radhakrishnan, S. 2007. 'The Legal Dimensions', *Seminar on Reproductive Health, Rights and Miscarriages: Problems & Solutions, 3 July 2007.* Hospital Tuanku Ja'afar, Seremban, Negeri Sembilan, Malaysia.

Raj, R., H. L. Chee and S. Rashidah. 1998. 'Between Modernization and Patriarchal Revivalism: reproductive negotiations among women in Peninsular Malaysia', in R.P. Petchesky and K. Judd (eds), *Negotiating Reproductive Rights: Women's Perspectives Across Countries and Cultures.* New York: Zed Books, pp. 108–144.

Rashidah Abdullah, F. 2007. 'In-Patient Management: Problems/constraints', *Seminar on Reproductive Health, Rights and Miscarriages: Problems & Solutions, 3 July 2007.* Hospital Tuanku Ja'afar, Seremban, Negeri Sembilan, Malaysia.

Rashidah Abdullah, R. 2000. 'Reproductive Health and Reproductive Rights: An Overview', in Zainah Anwar and Rashidah Abdullah (eds), *Islam, Reproductive Health and Women's Rights.* Kuala Lumpur: Sisters in Islam.

RRAAM. 2007a. *Survey Findings of Knowledge and Attitudes of Doctors and Nurses on Abortion by the Reproductive Rights Advocacy Alliance Malaysia* (RRAAM), unpublished.

———. 2007b. *Draft Position Paper of the Reproductive Rights Advocacy Alliance Malaysia* (RRAAM). Kuala Lumpur.

Shoba, A. 2007. 'Experiences in Reproductive Health among Women in the Shelter', *Seminar on Reproductive Health, Rights and Miscarriages: Problems & Solutions, 3 July 2007.* Hospital Tuanku Ja'afar, Seremban, Negeri Sembilan, Malaysia.

Sisters in Islam. 1998. *Public Forum on Contraception and Abortion jointly organised with The National Family Development and Population Board and ARROW.* Kuala Lumpur.

Siti Fathilah Kamaluddin 1997. 'Cultural Constructions of Abortion'. *Akademika* 51 (July): 77– 93.

———. 1998. 'Urban Malaysian Women's Experiences of Abortion: Some Implications for Policy', *Kajian Malaysia* (*Journal of Malaysian Studies*) 16 (1–2): 53–77.

UNFPA. 1994. *Programme of Action.* International Conference on Population and Development. UNFPA: New York.

WHO. 2003. *Safe Abortion. Policy and Technical Guidance for Health Systems.* WHO: Geneva.

Yut-Lin Wong, Y. L. 2003. 'Women's Access to Sexual Reproductive Health Services: Case Study of Kelantan Family Planning Association', in ARROW (ed), *Women's Access to Sexual Reproductive Health.* Kuala Lumpur: ARROW.

———. 2007. 'Women's Perspectives', *Seminar on Reproductive Health, Rights and Miscarriages: Problems & Solutions, 3 July 2007.* Hospital Tuanku Ja'afar, Seremban, Negeri Sembilan, Malaysia.

Chapter Ten

IMPROVING ACCESS TO SAFE TERMINATION OF PREGNANCY IN THAILAND

AN ANALYSIS OF POLICY DEVELOPMENTS FROM 1999 TO 2006

Nongluk Boonthai, Sripen Tantivess, Viroj Tangcharoensathien and Kamheang Chaturachinda

Unsafe abortions, especially those performed by non-health personnel, have long been a notable health problem in Thailand. The Thai Criminal Code of 1957 restricted the legal termination of pregnancy to cases where a woman's physical health was at risk or the pregnancy was due to rape.[1] Other potential indications for therapeutic abortion, such as a woman's mental health, foetal health conditions such as severe congenital malformations, or socioeconomic aspects, were not legally permitted. This resulted in painful dilemmas for women and medical staff, and contributed to unsafe abortion, mortality, morbidity and long-term negative consequences for Thai women and their families. Throughout the 1980s and 1990s, efforts to amend the law to broaden the definition of health and permit other clinical indications for the medical termination of pregnancies consistently failed, following concerted resistance from various groups. However, in 2005, a significant legal change in abortion practice was introduced when the Thai Medical Council issued its regulation on the conditions for medical practitioners to perform therapeutic termination of pregnancy in accordance with the Criminal Code. This included the extension of legitimised indications for physician-provided induced abortions to cover the mental health of the mother, and pregnancy-related stress in women in cases of high risk of hereditary diseases and congenital anomaly in their foetuses.

This chapter reviews the processes behind the issuance of the Medical Council's Regulation in 2005, by analysing the roles of key stakeholders, the influence of the local and international policy context, as well as the contents and the processes through which the new policy was developed. The anticipated evolution of the regulation and its ability to reduce unsafe abortions when it gets implemented is also discussed. To garner the information for this chapter, qualitative approaches were used, including documentary analysis. Semi-structured interviews with people involved in the policy process were also conducted, in order to provide a 'behind the scenes' view of so-called 'bottom-up' policy reform.

The Struggle for Legal Amendment: the Power of Discourses

As in many other countries, public policy regarding induced abortions, even those with a therapeutic purpose, is politically sensitive in Thailand. Prior to 2005, the issue of intentional pregnancy termination and the different policy alternatives available to facilitate it, repeatedly rose onto the political agenda in Thailand. One of the measures proposed by networks of non-government organisations (NGOs) including feminist and human rights groups, individual academics, lawyers, health professionals, social workers and journalists, was to amend the Criminal Code of 1957 to allow abortions performed by medical practitioners under extended conditions (Archavanitkul and Tharawan 2005). In 1981, proponents of such reform succeeded in passing a bill to amend the law through the House of Representatives (Intaraprasert and Boonthai 2005). However, owing to a vociferous public campaign by an anti-abortion coalition led by *Phalang Tham,* a popular religion-based political party, the bill failed to pass the Senate and policy reform efforts stalled.

Despite the unsuccessful reform movement, the period between 1970 and 1999 saw critical public debate among the advocates and opponents of such policy proposals. Due to intense lobbying by anti-abortionists, abortion came to be perceived by policy-makers, parliament members, and the general public as a socially disapproved act which would destroy morals, culture and the religion of the nation (Jantajamnong 1982 quoted in Whittaker 2004:26). The Buddhist prohibition of human and animal slaughter was evoked, and pregnancy termination was portrayed as a serious Buddhist sin or demerit akin to 'killing innocent children' or 'baby murder' (Whittaker 2004). Such representations affected the attitudes towards intentionally terminating gestations among the general public, but also specifically medical practitioners who were expected to provide safe abortion services under legal conditions. The accusation that reform would lead to 'free abortion' (in Thai, *'tham thang seri'*) became a common argument against any efforts to introduce reforms during two decades of debate. It became linked in discourse with the term 'free sex', suggesting that abortion reform would encourage promiscuity and deviant sexualities.

Despite arguments by opponents, different rhetoric was employed by reformists. The proponent coalitions asserted that legal amendment would be the only way to save the lives of a large number of 'unfortunate' women who died due to illegal abortion practice (Archavanitkul and Tharawan 2005). Corresponding research findings disseminated through the media were aimed at drawing the attention of government and the public to illegal abortion by emphasising its substantial magnitude and the plight of 'underprivileged' people. Human rights discourse entered the debate stressing 'women's rights over their bodies', a 'woman's rights to choose' and a 'family's liberty' to counter the anti-abortion campaigns. A number of feminist activists and academics argued that, because it was the right of people to control what develops in and happens to their bodies, women should be allowed to make their own decisions to maintain or terminate a pregnancy. They suggested that a husband and wife should have liberty to decide about the readiness of their family to have and nurture children.

When the HIV epidemic (MAP 2001) in Thailand significantly expanded to reach endemic proportions in the late 1980s, the disease moved from limited high-risk groups including male homosexuals, injecting drug users and commercial sex workers, to afflict the general population through sexual transmission. A significant increase in the number of HIV-positive housewives and children ignited further debate concerning the termination of pregnancy in infected mothers (Whittaker 2004). Some health professionals and politicians again proposed a legal amendment in 1995, proposing 'the tendency of malformation or serious diseases of the foetus' be included as an additional indicator for legal abortion (CDC Department 1995). The focus was placed on the definition of 'health': whether this term covered physical and mental health as well as the social well-being of pregnant women as stated in the World Health Organization (WHO) Constitution, or whether it was confined to the notion of physical health as generally perceived in Thai law. Some abortion advocates pointed out that realising the likelihood that their babies may be born with an incurable, fatal disease such as HIV could cause tremendous stress to the mothers[2], and therefore, termination of pregnancy should be allowed if the mothers so desired. It was suggested that the term 'health' in the legislation needed to be defined clearly for medical practitioners. After several requests to different authoritative bodies for clarification, in 1998 the Council of State ruled that the term 'health' referred solely to physical health, and that a provision to allow therapeutic abortions on the grounds of the mental health of the mothers would be uncontrollable. The Council of State also confirmed the illegality of the termination of pregnancy on the grounds of HIV.

New Millennium, New Approaches and Policy Shifts

The true power in driving public policies is the power to frame issues. Irrespective of how one organises the movement, if policy proposals run contra to people's beliefs by proposing solutions to which the public' does not want to listen, then those proposals are bound to fail. Therefore, the most crucial power is the power to define the issues. This is confirmed by the success of the pro-life network in Thailand; this group constructs the term 'abortion' as 'manslaughter', and the most awful instance of manslaughter as when a 'mother kills her own child' (Archavanitkul and Tharawan 2005:9). As a feminist activist from the NGO Foundation for Women suggested, 'Many doctors can see the problem from a public health perspective. But whenever there is a movement for change, some people believe that the movement is for free abortion, and they can't accept it. If the health issue is used, there would be more understanding' (quoted in Whittaker 2004: 59).

Recognising that open discussion of this delicate matter would not succeed in the legal amendment, from the late 1990s onwards supporters of reform employed alternative 'underground' strategies such as lobbying key officials within ministries responsible for the issue (Whittaker 2002) and presenting research studies to reassure them that amending the law would not result in 'free abortion', but would instead make induced abortion safer and better regulated.

As noted earlier, in 1999 the Public Health Ministry's Department of Health (DOH), with financial support from the WHO, conducted a study to examine the magnitude and profile of induced abortion in 787 government hospitals throughout the country, and to make policy recommendations to reduce unsafe abortion (Warakamin, Boonthai and Tangcharoensathien 2004). The induced abortion rate was calculated at 19.5 per one thousand live births, and almost half of the cases were in women younger than twenty-five years old. According to interviews with 1,850 patients conducted as part of this study, socio-economic problems were the major reason for terminating the pregnancy. Thirty per cent of these abortions, most of which were performed by non-health professionals, had resulted in serious complications. Government physicians reported intra-uterine deaths and congenital anomalies as the most common indicators for termination of pregnancy. This survey recommended that the Public Health Ministry and the Medical Council pursue legal reforms in order to improve the safety of induced abortions.

The policy advocacy based on the results of this study was well planned. Between 2000 and 2006, responsible officials in the DOH's Reproductive Health Division convened a series of seminars and consultations among concerned stakeholders such as medical professionals, social workers, attorneys, judges, academics and NGO representatives, where research findings were presented and discussed (Boonthai 2006). This aimed not only to seek effective solutions, but also to devise appropriate strategies and approaches to policy change. These discussions reached a consensus that, since the Medical Council had a mandate to provide policy recommendations in relation to the health of the population, it should take a leading role in the law reforms, both in terms of the content and the process. According to an obstetric specialist, the Medical Council was considered the most appropriate agency to undertake this task because past experience suggested the high risk of policy failure when 'top-down' approaches were employed, i.e. attempts at reform took place at the national legislative/policy level such as in the parliament and ministry departments. As this key informant argued, 'bottom-up' interventions which began within the Medical Council and then expanded further to the higher-level authorities, were expected to be more effective in enacting the abortion law amendments.

It took almost five years for the Medical Council to finalise its regulation extending the indications for legally induced abortion to include therapeutic terminations (see Table 10.1). This was the first time physical and mental health problems of the mother, including those associated with the high risk of severe disability or genetic diseases in the foetus, were clearly stated as the conditions for therapeutic abortion in accordance with the Criminal Law.

Table 10.1: Key content of the Medical Council's 'Regulation on Criteria for Performing Therapeutic Termination of Pregnancy in accordance with Section 305 of the Criminal Code', 2005.

- The therapeutic termination of pregnancy in accordance with Section 305 of the Criminal Code shall be performed only with the consent of the pregnant woman.
- The physician who performs the therapeutic termination of pregnancy has to be a medical practitioner, as defined by the Medical Professional Act.
- The therapeutic termination of pregnancy in accordance with Section 305 (1) of the Criminal Code shall be performed on the following conditions:
  (a) In case of necessity due to the physical health problem of the pregnant woman or;
  (b) In case of necessity due to the mental health problem of the pregnant woman, which has to be certified or approved by at least one medical practitioner other than the one who will perform the medical termination of pregnancy. In the case of severe stress due to the finding that the foetus has, or has a high risk of having, severe disability, or has, or has a high risk of having severe genetic disease, after the mother has been examined and received genetic counselling and the aforementioned matters have been acknowledged in writing by at least one medical practitioner other than the one who will perform the medical termination of pregnancy, the said pregnant woman shall be regarded as having a mental health problem as defined in (b) above.
- The therapeutic termination of pregnancy shall be performed as appropriate in a government hospital or government agency that provides overnight admission service to patients, or a medical infirmary that has beds for patients for overnight stay. A medical clinic is allowed to perform therapeutic termination of pregnancy only in cases when the gestational age is not over twelve weeks.

Source: Thai Medical Council 2005

Matters of 'Health' and Other Concerns

The Medical Council began working in February 2001, by firstly appointing a task group to formulate the strategic direction for the amendment of the Criminal Code, Article 305. This task group was chaired by the Secretary General of the Medical Council and consisted of representatives from: the Royal Colleges of Obstetricians,

Paediatricians, and Psychologists; the President of the Medical Genetics Association of Thailand; the Attorney General; the Secretary General of the Council of State; the Presidents of the National Council of Women and the National Commission on Human Rights; and experts in law, forensic medicine, as well as representatives from feminist groups (Thai Medical Council 2001).

At the same time, the Medical Council requested that the Royal Institute officially define the term 'health'.[3] As many had anticipated, a broad definition beyond the physical status of individuals and referring also to mental health, was suggested by the Royal Institute (Na Nagara 2001). Moreover, the Royal Institute argued that in the case of a pregnant woman, the notion of 'women's health' would also refer to the health of foetus, since the foetus was part of its mother. With a now clear explanation of this previously ambiguous terminology, in May 2001 the task group noted that it would not be necessary to modify any clauses of the 1957 Criminal Code. Rather, it was suggested that the Medical Council could issue a professional regulation on induced abortion as guidelines for medical practitioners to follow. As shown in notes from a Task Group meeting, the justification for this decision was that

> ... in order to pursue a rapid and timely drafting process, the Medical Council has to move its regulation forward. It is unnecessary to wait for the revision of the Criminal Code Article 305 by the Council of State. The Medical Council's Regulation can be used not only as practical guidelines for physicians, but also as legal reference for lawyers and others.... This would be better than leaving medical practitioners to provide abortion without direction and standard guidelines. (Drafting Group of the Medical Council's Regulation on Therapeutic Abortion 2002a)

Nevertheless, the task group members were aware that this regulation could not replace or overrule the existing Criminal Code, as the scope of enforcement of the Medical Council was limited to the ethical dimension of medical professional practice only. However, such a regulation, as a code of professional conduct, might be taken into account by the courts of justice if appropriate circumstances arose.

In early 2002, a new drafting group comprising experts in obstetrics, psychology, medical genetics, and laws, chaired by the Secretary General of the Medical Council, was appointed to devise the regulation. Most of these clinical experts were formally nominated as representatives of corresponding Royal Colleges or specialist associations. An official of the DOH and two lawyers from the Medical

Council served as the task group's Secretariat. Although the difficulties in defining 'health' were dealt with in the first phase of the Task Group, the further work of the Medical Council was not easy. From February 2002 until the regulation was enacted in December 2005, the centre of debate shifted to the definitions of the expanded indications for therapeutic abortion, namely 'mental health problems' of the mothers and 'congenital, heredity diseases' of the foetuses.

Since the indications for therapeutic abortion in accordance with the Criminal Code included only the health problems of the pregnant woman, the task group decided to consider the foetus' pathology only as the potential cause of mental distress in their mothers. The clinical criteria of the ICD10 were adopted to diagnose the mental health problems in the mothers; however, throughout 2002 and 2003, the indicators to be used for foetal disorders were not clearly defined (Drafting Group of the Medical Council's Regulation on Therapeutic Abortion 2003). The severity of health problems in the offspring was emphasised as inextricably linked to the determination of mental distress in pregnant women. The major concerns of the task group members included the possible abuse of the professional guidelines, which might encourage the provision of abortions by some physicians. In particular, there was a fear the Medical Council Regulation would be misconstrued and misunderstood by the general public. One of the task group members argued that, 'the introduction of ICD10 and tough criteria would restrain the public attitude that we promote free abortion' (Drafting Group of the Medical Council's Regulation on Therapeutic Abortion 2002b).

A further contentious issue was the question of who should approve or disapprove abortion in particular cases. While the task group agreed to have well-trained psychiatrists and specialists in medical genetics on call to make the decisions on the appropriateness of abortion on a case-by-case basis, they had to think about the practicality of such an option, since the personnel required were very small in number and concentrated in some areas, particularly in Bangkok and a few cities. This would make therapeutic abortion impossible in most parts of the country (Drafting Group of the Medical Council's Regulation on Therapeutic Abortion 2005). As a consequence, strict criteria and decision-making procedures for identifying the cases eligible for therapeutic termination of pregnancy were discussed back and forth within the task group and also at the higher-level committee of the Medical Council. The extensive time spent on consultations undertaken by the medical professional body during this period stemmed from their attempts to prevent potentially undesirable consequences, and also to ensure the practical and equitable access to medical termination of pregnancy across different geographical regions.

Policy Development Behind Closed Doors

In addition to addressing the contentious term of 'health' and developing criteria for eligible case identification, a key feature of the process to devise the Medical Council's Regulation on Therapeutic Termination of Pregnancy was that no activities carried out by the two task groups, the Medical Council, and concerned stakeholders were publicised. In addition, the number of actors involved in the consultations and decision-making were intentionally contained.

As mentioned earlier, in the early 2000s the law reform advocates realised the need to change the strategies they had been using to date, to place greater emphasis on lobbying particular policy-makers and other key players, while making use of empirical evidence to inform policy changes in order to reduce illegal abortions. The media was asked for cooperation only when education campaigns were developed to convey certain messages, focusing on the consequences of unsafe abortions and on the reproductive rights of women. The containment of public information could be observed throughout the period between 2001 and 2005, when the Medical Council's Regulation on Therapeutic Abortion was drafted. Although the drafting task group members considered that dissemination of the information on the current action of the Medical Council was necessary to counter the notion of 'free abortion promotion' and also to avoid misunderstanding in the public, key participants in this regulatory development process maintained in interviews in 2006 that they did not wish to convene media conferences on the work of the Medical Council's task groups (Drafting Task Group of the Medical Council Regulation on Therapeutic Abortion 2002; 2003).

Seminars and workshops on induced-abortion issues held by the DOH's Reproductive Health Division in collaboration with the Medical Council during this five-year period were aimed at consulting with certain groups of stakeholders such as medical practitioners, judges, lawyers, health administrators, representatives from Royal Medical Colleges, and parliament members (Boonthai 2006). Comments and recommendations obtained through these consultations were summarised and fed into the drafting process of the Regulation. Apart from this, particular people such as members of parliament, law experts, women's group leaders and board members of the Medical Council were invited to attend the task group meetings on some occasions (Drafting Group of the Medical Council's Regulation on Therapeutic Abortion 2004). This tactic was aimed at keeping these decision-makers and opinion leaders informed about the principles and details of all the issues, decisions and justifications discussed within the drafting group.

The Political Context of the Policy Innovation

The drafting process of the Medical Council's Regulation was well organised; however, not all activities ran smoothly without opposition and impediments. An analysis conducted by Whittaker (2002) suggests that there was political pressure from powerful politicians including the Health Minister against such reform, even though key persons in the anti-abortion alliance of the 1980s, especially General Chamlong Srimuang, the founder and head of *Phalang Tham*, a popular religious-based party, had left the political arena. The persistence of close relationship between the old politicians and new administration continued to affect abortion politics. As Whittaker (2002: 50) notes,

> Reformists still face the political problem that the present Prime Minister, Thaksin Shinawatra was a former leader of *Phalang Tham*. Although Chamlong Srimuang is no longer politically active, ... it is believed that he remains influential behind the scenes and is likely to have influence over the present PM. More significantly, the present Minister of Public Health, Sudarat Keyuraphan, is a former member of *Phalang Tham*. Any recommendations for amendments to the legislation would require her approval before being passed to parliament.

Such observation is confirmed by a number of key informants in this study. Despite the fact that the Medical Council was an independent, professional authority, ostensibly outside the command line of the Health Ministry, the Secretariat of the task group for drafting the Medical Council's regulation was partially composed of officials from the DOH's Reproductive Health Division. It was revealed in interviews conducted in 2006 that there were attempts made by the Minister and also health administrators at the ministerial and departmental level to hinder the abortion law amendments, including the formulation of the Medical Council's regulation. It is noteworthy that some of these senior medical officials, even some Board members of the professional authority, personally opposed the role of medical practitioners in providing abortion service. As argued by interviewees, this resulted in the significant delay of formal communication and bureaucratic procedure within the Public Health Ministry and between the Ministry and the Medical Council.

Although the law amendment advocates attempted to control information about the development of the Medical Council's Regulation, in some instances information was disclosed to the public. In response, anti-abortion campaigns emerged in the media, appearing on the front pages of newspapers. Sensational cases described women as 'fun-loving, morally corrupt' students whose babies' remains were discovered in illegal abortion clinics (Whittaker 2002: 50). These articles not only stirred public opposition to any means to deal with unwanted pregnancy, but also encouraged the Health Minister to present her strong position to harshly penalise abortion providers and women who had abortions. Fortunately, when the Medical Council's Regulation on Therapeutic Abortion was passed from the professional authority to be endorsed by the Health Minister, there had been changes to the cabinet: Sudarat Keyuraphan was replaced by a professor of respiratory medicine whose standpoint towards therapeutic termination of pregnancy was unclear. Eventually, the Deputy Health Minister, who had no opposition to such issues at all, approved the Medical Council's Regulation.

The international environment had a relatively minor and indirect influence on the abortion policy shift in Thailand. For example, the WHO country budget supported the national survey of unsafe abortion in 1999 (Warakamin et al. 2004), the Planned Parenthood Federation of America International supported the development of curriculum for a training course in safe abortion for physicians and nurses in 2004–2005, and WHO also supported the workshops and meetings in the movement towards amendment of related regulations. Although the global frameworks on women's rights and reproductive health had long been established and adopted by Thai policy makers and responsible agencies (for example, ICPD helped put reproductive health programs high on the policy agenda in the Ministry of Public Health) some elements of global frameworks, such as the liberty to discontinue gestations and access to safe abortion service, were neglected. However, the recommendations, practice guidelines, education and information materials, networks and activities developed internationally have inspired and indirectly supported the movement of Thai safe-abortion advocates to some extent. For instance, a key informant pointed out the following:

> I attended international conferences several times, from which I learned about problems and strategies that were employed in other countries. Discussion and comments made in these meetings reflected the true impediments. Crucially, the term 'health' as stated by abortion laws, similar to what people perceive, refers to only physical well being. Even physicians usually argue for the narrow definition. Actually, they understand the true meaning ... but they just don't want to provide abortion. This is the weak point we have to address. (Interview, 2006)

The Way Forward

After the enactment of the Medical Council's Regulation, a number of activities have been undertaken by, among others, the DOH's Reproductive Health Division, the Royal Thai College of Obstetricians & Gynaecologists, the Medical Council and the Women's Health and Reproductive Rights Foundation of Thailand, with technical support from experts from teaching hospitals in different regions. Most activities involved information and training programmes for physicians and nurses. The objectives of these programmes were to build up the providers' capacity in performing safe abortion and related services such as providing pre- and post-abortion counselling, contraception, and family planning to women with therapeutic needs (Boonthai 2006). They also aimed to improve the poor attitudes of practitioners towards abortion practice. Nevertheless, responsible officials and experts admitted in interviews that this is difficult to achieve, since it depends a great deal on the training and socialisation that occurred when these personnel studied in medical schools.

Public advocacy and education work by the The Women's Health and Reproductive Rights Foundation of Thailand (WHRRF) continues. On 20–23 January 2010, the 1st International Congress on Women's Health and Unsafe Abortion (IWAC 2010) was held at the at the Imperial Queens Park Hotel in Bangkok. This public event was organized by the WHRRF (primary organizers included authors Nongluk Boonthai and Kamhaeng Chaturachinda). The idea was mooted in 2007 and members of the Foundation lobbied to garner support to hold a congress specifically devoted to highlight the issue of abortion. A broad alliance, including the with the Department of Health, Ministry of Health, The Royal Thai College of Obstetricians and Gynaecologists, College of Public Health Sciences, Chulalongkorn University, Faculty of Public Health, Mahidol University, and

DOCUMENT 10.1. The Bangkok Declaration 2010 on Women's Health and Unsafe Abortion, Bangkok, IWAC, 23 January 2010

We participants, from a wide range of health professionals of more than 62 nations across the globe at the First IWAC 2010, declared the following:

We believe that:

- Unsafe abortion is both a public health and a women's rights issue.
- Every woman should have a free choice over whether to continue her pregnancy or to terminate it.
- A safe and appropriate method of termination of pregnancy should be made available to every woman requesting to end a pregnancy.
- A new approach should be initiated in countries where the "abortion related laws" are rigid and ignore the fundamental rights of women.

We understand that:

- All women, especially teens and adolescents need to receive clear and accurate information and knowledge about basic reproduction and reproductive health issues to avoid unintended pregnancies.
- Unsafe abortion is completely preventable provided societies decide to do so. The most effective way to prevent unsafe abortion is to provide safe abortion services. This has been documented in those countries where abortion was legalized and accessible.

We call on:

- All developed and developing countries,to work hand in hand, to provide techniques, regulations and funding to eliminate unsafe abortions.
- Women's groups and NGOs working for women's health to empower women to achieve gender equality in society.
- All governments should pay more attention to the issue of unsafe abortion.
- All governments should significantly increase funding to prevent unsafe abortion.

We encourage:

- All countries experiencing unsafe abortion to work together and learn from each other's approach to tackling the issue.
- Those countries which have been successful in reducing unsafe abortion to share and/or disseminate their experiences with other countries.

We respect:

- The rights of each individual woman to access ***safe*** abortion care.

the Population and Community Development Association and others supported the event. It was endorsed by International Federation of Obstetrics and Gynaecology (FIGO) and Asia Oceania Federation of Obstetrics and Gynecology (AOFOG). In a demonstration of the political success of their advocacy efforts, the congress was opened by the Prime Minister of Thailand, The Right Honorable Mr. Abhisit Vejjajiva, MP. It was attended by 348 international delegates from 64 nations and 220 local participants. The congress aimed to provide a scientific platform to highlight the universal problem of unsafe abortion as a public health issue and one of women's health and rights. It highlighted the advances and current safe abortion technology being used in the developed world and provided an opportunity for global networking. The Bangkok Declaration, endorsed by delegates on the final day of proceedings signals a new openness and determination by reproductive rights advocates in Thailand to confront this issue and advocate for further change.

Discussion

In order to tackle the problem of unsafe abortion, comprehensive and wide-ranging strategies are required, ranging from health promotion, to prevention of unwanted pregnancies, to enhancement of access to quality health services. Multi-disciplinary approaches, not only clinically oriented, are indispensable in this process. The Bangkok Declaration 2010 is a clear statement of the needs of countries to address the issue of unsafe abortion and for advocates to share and support our efforts.

The modification of abortion legislation is highly political and setting specific. In contrast to the Thai example discussed in this chapter, for instance, the success in introducing abortion law amendment in Guyana during the 1990s was encouraged by the openness of the reform process: the movement to support the new law was organised through the media, educating all interested parties including the public about the morbidity and mortality associated with illegal abortion, the weaknesses of existing 'prohibitive' abortion regulation, and the potential effectiveness of the legislation permitting therapeutic abortion in improving women's health (Nunes and Delph 1995).

The extension of the definition for allowing therapeutic abortion through the development of the Thai Medical Council's Regulation in 2005 can be regarded as a result of strategic management: the whole process to make such policy change was carefully planned and organised. The long-term unsuccessful struggle to amend the Criminal Code during the previous phase encouraged the law reform advocates to try a new 'bottom-up' approach, addressing the issue through the medical profession, instead of direct lobbying of politicians and legislators.

Policy-analysis frameworks and models may be helpful in understanding why this tactic worked. Walt and Gilson (1994) suggest the development and implementation of public policies results from interactions between three elements: actors, process, and context. Actors, as groups and individuals, pursue their interests by exercising power over others (Walt 1994). Those who are influential are able to lead the process, manipulate the policies, and gain benefits.

In some instances, power is conceptualised as 'thought control'. As Lukes has pointed out, 'power is the ability to shape meanings and perceptions of reality which might be done through the control of information, the mass media and/or through controlling the processes of socialization' (1974 quoted in Buse et al. 2005: 23). Such a notion of power helps explain why the Thai safe-abortion advocates failed to make changes in legislation prior to 2001. This is in line with the argument of women's rights coalition leaders:

> The true power in driving public policies is the power to frame problematic issues. Irrespective of how we organise the campaigns – if we promote the policy proposals which conflict with people's belief, that is, propose solutions which the public doesn't want to listen to, our movement will always fail.... The most crucial power is the power to define the issues. The Pro-Life network succeeds because they construct the term 'abortion' as 'manslaughter' – the most awful manslaughter is 'mother kills her own child'(sic) in such a case. (Archavanitkul and Tharawan 2005: 9)

Several political strategies are suggested for policy change. Among others, Roberts and colleagues maintain that the feasibility of facilitating policy innovation can be enhanced by strategically managing the position, power, players and perception (2004 quoted in Buse et al. 2005: 182). Given that the reformist networks realised that they were unable to convince the opposition and then obtain support from the general public, they opted to alter their policy proposal by emphasising the regulation which would affect only medical practitioners. In addition, the suppression of information on what was carried out by the Medical Council and its specialist Task Group was another measure aimed at allowing discussion of reforms to take place without generating a sensationalist public debate. Meanwhile, by organising presentations and discussions on the magnitude of unsafe abortion and policy alternatives among some stakeholders such as physicians, members of legislative authorities, lawyers and NGOs, the Medical Council could be seen as distributing political assets to potential supporters for policy changes.

This chapter illustrates the Thai experience to extend the legal conditions under which therapeutic abortion could be performed by medical practitioners. It sheds some light on the political tactics employed by reformists, including managing the scope of policy proposals and involvement of selected stakeholders, after repeated past failures in campaigning for amendment of the Criminal Law. The issuance of the Medical Council's Regulation on Therapeutic Termination of Pregnancy, which included a clear, broadened definition of 'mother's health', was a step forward in making abortion service more accessible among Thai women. However, to what extent this policy will be implemented and beneficial to the real target groups such as mothers with low socio-economic status, pregnancy resulting from contraceptive failure, and those infected with HIV, remains a crucial question (Whittaker 2002).

The different barriers to abortion services on both the demand and supply sides of the equation, need to be adequately addressed. The situation in South Africa offers an example of inappropriately dealing with such barriers: although medical abortion has been legalised since 1997, women in rural areas face notable access difficulties due to inadequate distribution of relevant information and prohibitive travelling costs (Cooper et al. 2005).

Thai activists also recognised that the attitudes of physicians and paramedics against induced abortion could not be modified by introducing regulatory intervention alone. Considerable need exists among providers for training on counselling, the use of medicines and equipment in inducing abortion and for the treatment of complications (Billing et al. 2002).

Ultimately, however, the true barrier to safe abortion in most settings is the negative perceptions of people in broader society. As Berer (2002: 3) has asserted:

> Abortion is not just illegal and clandestine insofar as the law is concerned, but also in people's minds. Until a society accepts that abortion is needed by women and that women and abortion providers

should not be punished for it, legal abortions will rarely be provided except in exceptional circumstances.

Acknowledgements

We acknowledge the significant contribution Professor Pramuan Virutamasen on behalf of the Thai Medical Council, members of the Council and the Royal Thai College of Obstetricians and Gynaecologists in the process of the legislation reform and improving safe abortion service in Thailand. Activities of the project on improved access to safe abortion were partially supported by World Health Organization and Planned Parenthood Federation of America-International.

Notes

1. Under Section 305 of the 1957 Criminal Code, abortion is allowed if performed by medical practitioner and necessary for a woman's health, or because the pregnancy is due to offences such as rape, seduction of a girl under age fifteen, fraud, deceit, violence, etc. in the procuration or seduction (The Population Council 1981).
2. Note that effective interventions to prevent vertical transmission of HIV were not available at that time, thus the chance of a newborn getting the virus from its parents was high: more than 23 per cent of vertical transmission.
3. The Royal Institute is an autonomous government agency, founded in 1933. It acts as a consultant and advisory body on academic matters, as requested by the government.

References

Archavanitkul, K. and T. Kanokwan. 2005. 'Movement for Abortion Rights', in *Women Care in Relation to Abortion*. Khon Kaen: Department of Health, Division of Reproductive Health.

Berer, M. 2002. 'Making Abortion a Woman's Right Worldwide', *Reproductive Health Matters* 10 (19): 1–8.

Billing, D. L., C. Moreno, C. Ramos, D. Gonzalez de Leon, R. Ramirez, L. Villasenor Martinez and M. Rivera Diaz. 2002. 'Constructing Access to Legal Abortion Services in Mexico City', *Reproductive Health Matters* 10 (19): 86–94.

Boonthai, N. 2006. 'Summary of the Project to Prevent Mortality due to Unsafe Abortion and the Development of the Medical Council Regulation on Therapeutic Termination of Pregnancy in Accordance with the Criminal Code Article 305, 2005'. Nonthaburi: Department of Health, Reproductive Health Division.

Communicable Disease Control Department. 1995. Official letter from the CDC Department to the Medical Council. Nonthaburi: Ministry of Public Health.

Cooper, D., K. Dickson, K. Blanchard, L. Cullingworth, N. Mavimbela, C. Mollendorf, L. van Bogaert, L. and B. Winikoff. 2005. 'Medical Abortion: The Possibilities for Introduction in the Public Sector in South Africa', *Reproductive Health Matters* 13 (26): 35–43.

Drafting Group of the Medical Council's Regulation on Therapeutic Abortion. 2002a. Record of Meeting 1/2002, February 21, 2002. Nonthaburi: The Medical Council of Thailand.

———. 2002b. *Record of Meeting 3/2002, December 2, 2002.* Nonthaburi: The Medical Council of Thailand.

———. 2003. *Record of Meeting 1/2003, December 22, 2003.* Nonthaburi: The Medical Council of Thailand.

———. 2004. *Record of Meeting 4/2004, July 29, 2004.* Nonthaburi: The Medical Council of Thailand.

———. 2005. *Record of Meeting 1/2005, April 4, 2005.* Nonthaburi: The Medical Council of Thailand.

Intaraprasert, S. and N. Boonthai. 2005. 'Challenge for Unsafe Abortion', *Journal of Medical Association of Thailand* 88 (Suppl 2): S104–S107.

Jantajamnong, S. 1982. *Abortion and medical and social problems.* Bangkok: Rug Reuang Sasana Phim.

Lukes, S. 1974. *Power: A Radical Approach.* London: Macmillan.

Medical Council. 2001. *The Medical Council Notification on the Appointment of the Subcommittee on the Amendment of the Criminal Code, Article 305, dated February 16, 2001.* Nonthaburi.

Monitoring the AIDS Pandemic (MAP) network. 2001. 'The status and trends of HIV/AIDS/STI epidemics in Asia and the Pacific', October 4, 2001. Retrieved 18 May 2007 from http://data.unaids.org/UNA-docs/map2001_en.doc

Na Nagara, P. 2001. *The Definition of 'Health', a letter dated February 27, 2001.* Bangkok: The Royal Institute, Science Division.

Nunes, F. E. and Y. M. Delph. 1995. 'Making Abortion Law Reform Happen in Guyana: A Success Story', *Reproductive Health Matters* November (6): 12–23.

Roberts, M. J., W. Hsiao, P. Berman and M. R. Reich. 2004. *Getting Health Reform Right. A Guide to Improving Performance and Equity.* Oxford: Oxford University Press.

Walt, G. 1994. *Health Policy: An Introduction to Process and Power.* London: Zed Books.

Walt, G. and L. Gilson. 1994. 'Reforming the health sector in developing countries: the central role of policy analysis', *Health Policy and Planning* 9 (4): 353–370.

Warakamin, S., N. Boonthai and V. Tangcharoensathien. 2004. 'Induced Abortion in Thailand: Current Situation in Public Hospitals and Legal Perspectives', *Reproductive Health Matters* 12 (24 supplement): 147–156.

Whittaker, A. 2002. 'The Struggle for Abortion Law Reform in Thailand', *Reproductive Health Matters* 10 (19): 15–53.

———. 2004. *Abortion, sin and the state in Thailand.* Abingdon: Routledge Curzon.

Chapter Eleven

EPILOGUE

FURTHER CHALLENGES

Andrea Whittaker

The study of abortion challenges us as researchers and advocates. This book strives to reflect current concerns in social science scholarship on abortion in Asia and consider the status of advocacy in the region. In this brief epilogue, I consider some of the contributions of this book to the study of reproduction more broadly and consider questions for further research.

The contributions of this book place abortion within the social management of fertility rather than situating it as a separate, extraordinary category. The various chapters remind us that abortion is not something divorced from gender relations, sexuality, marriage, family formation and fertility, but rather forms part of processes through which people shape and reshape their relationships and their families. The essays situate women's experiences within their families, social settings and institutions. They also bring out the centrality of gender and the need to consider the negotiations around power and agency in women and men's relationships and within families.

Although the accepted meanings of feminism in our different countries and cultural contexts may vary, the approaches within this book all display a common concern with the conditions of women and a commitment to transform gender oppression alongside the other systems of domination that divide women by class, race, ethnicity, religion and nationality. They highlight how states are involved in intimate interventions into the reproductive lives of their citizens and how women's bodies and experiences are structured by macro and micro relations of power, class and gender politics.

Common to the chapters are the negotiations over the definitions and understandings of abortion and the divisions that exist between ideology, practice and the law. In many places, understandings of early pregnancy as little more than a 'lump of blood' and the ubiquitous use of local hot herbal medicines and tonics throughout Asia 'to bring blood down' blur lines between natural abortion and induced abortions. In many cultures the 'quickening' or sense of foetal movement in the womb affirms pregnancy, a reminder of pregnancy as an embodied experience, not merely a laboratory test result. Yet throughout the region, the widespread availability of pregnancy tests, ultrasonography and other biomedical technologies are changing definitions and relationships to pregnancies. Laws regulating terminations now depend heavily upon biomedical definitions of pregnancy, gestation, foetal health and viability. Struggles over the medical profession's power to define and govern termination of pregnancy versus women's autonomy and rights to make such decisions run throughout this book.

The reader of this book is forced to confront the extreme poverty, marginality and structural violence experienced by many women and men in the region. The image of the couple willing to sell an eye each on the Burmese border in Belton's chapter, the woman begging for an abortion in a Dhaka slum described by Rashid, the couples struggling to borrow enough money for their abortion in Tamil Nadu described by Ramachandar and Pelto, speak of how unplanned pregnancy represents a crisis for many women, plunging a couple into debt and further poverty. The fact that economic reasons are rarely acceptable grounds for legal termination of pregnancy in many countries only serves to further victimise the most vulnerable.

The politics of abortion operates on both the local level, such as families' negotiations over pregnancies and money, or local clinics' refusals to treat women, but also at the state and international level. The last three chapters describe the political, religious and institutional complexities involved in attempts at legal reforms in Indonesia and Thailand and the implementation of policy in Malaysia. They remind us of the powerful political influence and rhetorical strategies of religious lobby groups, whether Buddhist, Muslim or Roman Catholic appealing to notions of distinct Asian family values, culture and religious ethics.

The chapters of this book demonstrate how qualitative methodologies can add great depth and compassion to our understanding of abortion and there remains a shortage of studies utilising rigorous ethnographic methods in Asia. Micro-level ethnographic detail can enhance our understanding of broader demographic and public health trends and economic decision-making in ways not possible through broad surveys and statistical analysis. Sensitive, in-depth interviews and participant observation allows us to enter others' experience. Yet some chapters raise epistemological questions regarding the difficulties of capturing the emotional experience of others on sensitive and private topics. How can one relay the significance of silences, minimal words, pauses and looks which may convey much yet always translate inadequately? How best do we explain the hidden narratives behind smiles and stock replies? Interviews may force explanations of previously secret knowledge, demanding levels of introspection, self-objectification and narrative closure that women and men may not have performed previously. The authors in this volume reinforce the need to respect the women and men with whom and of whom we speak and make problematic any simplistic interpretations of motives or categorisations of data.

The contributions display tensions between the different languages, styles and emphases across work written by academics, activists and the international NGO community. The positions entailed in the language used in abortion research are themselves worthy of study. The final chapters inspire the need to study the politics and processes of how reform and change within health systems takes place – an anthropology of activism. These chapters also demonstrate the need for advocates working within NGOS and health systems to have increased sensitivity to the reproductive politics of women's groups, national agendas and political histories in their work, and a diversity of strategies for implementing change.

Most contributors to this volume are only too aware of the politics of their own research and the texts and ethnographies they produce. A number of the contributors view themselves as 'scholar-activists'. They combine their research with advocacy work and see this as the only legitimate position for privileged researchers working on women's issues. Their work spurs us to consider the role of research in advocacy. We need to problematise the relationships we have with our informants, the political implications of our methods, the modes of presentation of our results, the influence of our funding sources and be conscious of the unequal relations of power they entail. Particularly for Western scholars of Asia, these are often uncomfortable questions. It is hoped that this volume will precipitate further collaborative ventures across the region, to strengthen advocacy on this issue in our respective countries and share our skills and experience.

An Agenda for Further Research

There remain a number of gaps in our understanding and questions not asked about the experience of abortion in Asia. By way of concluding this book, I suggest a number of topics for further research. All pose methodological and ethical challenges, but also opportunities to contribute significantly not only to our disciplines but to advocacy work.

The first set of issues involves the experiences of particularly vulnerable groups of people. The issue of HIV/AIDS and abortion remains a sensitive one across the region, as a number of countries face growing numbers of infected women, many of whom only learn of their infection when they present for antenatal care (de Bruyn 2003; Whittaker 2000). The legal frameworks in a number of countries in the region still make it illegal for a woman who is HIV positive to terminate her pregnancy. While the advent of new treatment regimes for pregnant women is greatly decreasing the risk of vertical transmission, the fact remains that many women dealing with such a diagnosis may choose not to continue a pregnancy, depending on their circumstances and emotional state. Similarly, those who do choose to continue their pregnancies may face pressure to terminate and encounter a lack of information, support and counselling about treatments. Although some participatory research with HIV positive groups has been undertaken, much more needs to be done to document this issue.

Silence also surrounds the issues of disability and abortion. Across Asia, people with disability suffer a variety of forms of discrimination, one of which is the neglect of all aspects of their sexuality and reproductive health. A number of issues deserve our attention. These include the experience of people with disabilities and pregnancy and pressures to abort; issues surrounding the forms of genetic counselling given to people carrying inheritable conditions; the growing use of ultrasound and various prenatal genetic diagnostic tests, their interpretation and the consequences for terminations.

Another group about whom little is known is the experience of adolescents seeking abortions, despite adolescents being a priority for research for a number of donors. Partly, this is due to the enormous difficulty in locating this population and the ethical difficulties in doing so, particularly for unmarried adolescents. Given the moral panic across Asia over earlier ages of initiation of sexual activity, and what is seen as modern Western values usurping Asian values, it is surprising that so little detailed work has been done of adolescents' experiences of abortion decision-making and experience of services. We especially know very little about the men involved in these relationships. Even in countries where abortion is legal under a range of situations, it is often restricted to married women. As Rashid's chapter in this book reminds us, adolescents are particularly vulnerable, often lacking power, finances and knowledge to determine the outcomes of their pregnancies, whether their desire is to continue them or terminate them. As Bennett's (2001) study in Indonesia notes, young women with unplanned premarital pregnancy face personal and familial shame, compromised marriage prospects, abandonment by their partners, single motherhood, a stigmatised child, early cessation of education, and an interrupted income or career. Given that most cultures in the region do not countenance children born out of wedlock, in the absence of an offer of marriage, single women in the region often have little choice but to resort to abortion. In India, girls and women often choose to end their own lives rather than continue socially unacceptable pregnancies (Ganatra 2003).

A further, often invisible and silenced group is that of migrants and displaced people in conflict zones (Lehmann 2002; Belton 2007; Belton and Whittaker 2007). Asia has the greatest proportion of displaced people in the world, and the issue of the reproductive health needs, including the need for access to abortion services for migrant and displaced people, remains one only recently attracting attention. Belton's chapter in this collection points to the need for more studies employing detailed ethnography to understand the experiences, practices and needs of these groups. Large numbers of displaced women and refugees experience rape or are at risk for pregnancy due to a lack of contraceptives. Similarly, women in conflict zones may be discouraged from using contraceptives due to inaccessibility or pronatalist nationalist ideologies. The numbers of such women dying from maternal related causes may not even be recognised or recorded if they are not citizens of the countries in which they find themselves (Belton and Whittaker 2007). The special needs of women in such circumstances needs to be recognised, and research is needed to address the question of most appropriate forms of service provision for mobile and disenfranchised groups.

Within all studies of abortion, there needs to be greater sensitivity to the linkages between violence, pregnancy and abortion. It is estimated by the WHO that globally, one in five women have been physically or sexually abused in their lifetime, usually by someone they know (1997 in Hessini 2004: 11). Violence may be associated with an inability to prevent unwanted pregnancies due to non-consensual sex, or may cause pregnancy loss or result in abortions due to the violent relationship, or being forced to abort. Having an abortion may also trigger domestic violence. Such violence may be compounded by the abuse of women who present for abortion related care (de Bruyn 2003b; see also Wu et al. 2005). We need to refine our methods for asking about violence and ensure that researchers do not avoid the issue for fear of the topic being 'too sensitive'. There is a need for systematic studies on violence and abortion if there is to be advocacy and improvement in services on this issue.

The effects of new technologies in reproductive regimes also requires interrogation. There have been few studies on reproductive technologies in Asia. Ultrasound technologies are becoming increasingly common in urban areas throughout Asia and have had a number of consequences for women's maternity care. One negative consequence of ultrasound has been its use to determine the sex of a foetus. Despite the illegality of the use of such technologies for prenatal sex screening in a number of countries, sex selective abortion remains a serious concern in India and China (see discussion in Miller 2001). Yet these technologies have had other less well recognised effects which warrant further investigation. Rashidah Abdullah and Yut-Lin Wong's paper on Malaysia note that the use of ultrasound pictures in pre-abortion counselling reassures Malay Muslim patients that their pregnancies are still 'lumps of blood' and hence permissible to abort within Islamic principles. As Gammeltoft notes in her chapter, the increased use of ultrasound also results in the identification of foetal malformations and the possibility for a termination of wanted pregnancies on medical grounds. Clearly, there is a need for more ethnographic research of the type undertaken by Gammeltoft to understand the ways in which ultrasound and other technologies such as amniocentesis are being used, interpreted and understood by women and their health providers and the implications for increased late terminations. This is especially important in countries such as Thailand, which have recently reformed their abortion regulations to include foetal malformations as legal grounds for abortion (see Nongluk Boonthai et al. this volume). Gammeltoft's chapter reminds us of how these technologies such as prenatal diagnosis and ultrasonography fundamentally alter knowledge about a pregnancy, making the invisible visible, with consequences for local perceptions of foetal moral status and ethical perceptions of abortion. She describes the phenomenology of therapeutic abortions, the ambivalent decisions that these technologies prompt and women's emotionally charged experience. Such technologies make choices possible but can increase woman's dependency on the knowledge and advice of experts. One might speculate as to the consequences as higher resolution ultrasonography becomes more widely available. The introduction of 3D and 4D imaging promises to further complicate ethical subjectivity. Finally, as noted in the overview, new abortion technologies, namely vacuum aspiration (MVA) and medication abortion, are being introduced in many Asian countries. These technologies are the recommended methods of abortion during the first trimester (World Health Organization 2003). Studies of what women want and prefer and the effect of these new technologies upon the practice and experience of abortion are needed.

A related issue urgently requiring investigation is the movement and trade in medication abortion drugs. There is a large unmet demand across Asia for effective means of abortion combined with largely unregulated trade across borders and poor pharmaceutical regulation in many countries. Just as patent menstrual regulators and contraceptives are traded across the region, anecdotal reports suggest Chinese abortion drugs are available on the Cambodian borders (Hoban pers. com.) and Indian abortion drugs may be available for private purchase in Nepal (Tamang and Tamang 2005). Ethnographic research is needed to explore this trade, how these drugs are used, whether they are used safely and by whom.

Finally, as noted earlier, there is a need for an anthropology of the struggles, social processes and groups through which abortion reform is contested in Asia. We need to understand not only the activists groups seeking reform but also those opposing it and the cultural discourses and narratives they draw upon in their campaigns for popular support. Such struggles take place in diverse ways and utilise a range of cultural, religious and legal frameworks to justify their positions.

The study of abortion requires a multilayered perspective that pays attention to reproductive practices, negotiations and resistances and their interconnections at a local and global level. It poses rich questions for the social sciences fundamentally concerned with agency and structure, gendered power relations, social inequalities, the governance of populations and global politics of reproduction. It demands engaged scholarship confronting an issue fundamental to women's rights across the region.

References

Belton, S. 2007. 'Borders of Fertility: Unplanned Pregnancy and Unsafe Abortion in Burmese Women Migrating to Thailand', *Health Care for Women International* 28: 419–433.

Belton, S. and A. Whittaker. 2007. 'Kathy Pan, Sticks and Pummelling: Techniques Used to Induce Abortion by Burmese Women on the Thai Border', *Social Science & Medicine* 65: 1512–1523.

Bennett, L. R. 2001. 'Single Women's Experiences of Premarital Pregnancy and Induced Abortion in Lombok, Eastern Indonesia', *Reproductive Health Matters* 9 (17): 37–43.

de Bruyn, M. 2003. 'Safe Abortion for HIV-Positive Women with Unwanted Pregnancy: A Reproductive Right', *Reproductive Health Matters* 11 (22): 152–161.

Ganatra, B. and S. Hirve. 2002. 'Induced Abortions among Adolescent Women in Rural Maharashtra, India', *Reproductive Health Matters* 10 (19): 76–85.

Hessini, L. 2004. *Advancing reproductive health as a human right: Progress toward safe abortion care in selected Asian countries since ICPD.* Chapel Hill, NC: Ipas.

Lehmann, A. 2002. 'Safe Abortion: A Right for Refugees?' *Reproductive Health Matters:* 151–155.

Miller, B. 2001. 'Female-selective abortion in Asia: Patterns, policies and debates', *American Anthropologist* 103 (4): 1083–1095.

Tamang, A. and J. Tamang. 2005. 'Availability and Acceptability of Medical Abortion in Nepal: Health Care Providers' Perspectives', *Reproductive Health Matters* 13 (26): 110–119.

Whittaker, A. 2000. 'Reproductive Health Rights and Women with HIV in Thailand', *Development Bulletin* 52 (June): 35–37.

World Health Organization. 2003. *Safe Abortion: Technical and Policy Guidance for Health Systems.* Geneva: World Health Organization.

Wu, J., S. Guo and C. Qu. 2005. 'Domestic Violence against Women Seeking Induced Abortion in China', *Contraception* 72: 117–121.

Glossary

Abortifacient: any substance that ends a pregnancy and causes an abortion.

Dilation and curettage (D&C): also known as 'sharp curettage', involves dilating the cervix with mechanical dilators or drugs and using sharp metal curettes to scrape the walls of the uterus. It is less safe than vacuum aspiration with higher risks of complications than vacuum aspiration and is more painful (WHO 2003: 34).

Induced abortion: an abortion that is brought about intentionally as opposed to a spontaneous abortion or miscarriage. Also called Termination of Pregnancy (TOP)

Kovac's procedure (modified): for second-trimester abortions between sixteen and twenty weeks since the last menstrual period (LMP). It involves the insertion of a condom-covered catheter to introduce an extra-amniotic saline infusion to induce contractions.

Manual Vacuum Aspiration (MVA): is a procedure using a syringe, valves and a plunger used for uterine aspiration. It can be used for first-trimester abortions, treatment of incomplete abortions and endometrial biopsies. It is portable and small and can be used in a variety of settings.

Medication abortion/medical abortion: the use of a pharmacological drug to terminate pregnancy, also called non-surgical abortion (WHO 2003: 23). Along with vacuum aspiration it is the WHO-recommended method of choice for early termination of pregnancy. Mifepristone followed by a prostaglandin has been demonstrated to be safe and effective up to nine completed weeks of pregnancy (WHO 2003: 30). The term 'medication abortion' is used in this book in preference to 'medical abortion' to avoid terminological confusion (see Wietz et al 2004).

Menstrual Regulation (MR): refers to methods used to ensure the resumption of menstruation. This may include the use of herbal and traditional means. The WHO (2003: 22) defines menstrual regulation as 'early uterine evacuation without laboratory or ultrasound confirmation of pregnancy for women who report delayed menses' and usually refers to procedures performed up to six weeks following the onset of the last menstrual period. Also sometimes termed menstrual extraction.

Post-Abortion Care (PAC): According to the Postabortion Care Consortium (2002), the five essential elements of post-abortion care include counselling to identify and respond to women's emotional and physical health needs and other concerns; treatment of incomplete and unsafe abortion and complications; contraceptive and family planning; and reproductive and other health services provided on-site or via referrals; and community and service provider partnerships for prevention and mobilization of resources.

Unsafe abortion: a procedure for terminating an unwanted pregnancy either by persons lacking the necessary skills or in an environment lacking the minimal medical standards or both (WHO 2003: 12)

Index